Why Raise Ugly Kids?

Why Raise Ugly Kids?

FULFILL YOUR CHILD'S HEALTH AND HAPPINESS POTENTIAL

Hal A. Huggins, DDS

With a foreword by
Lendon Smith, MD

ARLINGTON HOUSE PUBLISHERS
Westport, Connecticut

Thanks to the Price-Pottenger Foundation for the use of their photographs; Price-Pottenger Foundation, Box 2614, La Mesa, CA 92041.

And a special acknowledgment to those people who spent so much time assisting me in gathering specialized information. They include: Den and Barb Michael for Indian information; Wade Webster for molding the clay heads; Karl Nishimuri, D.D.S., for introducing me to X-ray techniques that show facial distortion; Michael Hoffman, M.D., who showed the anthropologic aspects of skulls; Robert Kernott, D.D.S., for his work in three-dimensional analysis of the skull which showed the actual changes when sleeping habits were changed; Fred Feiler, M.D., for his support from the field of orthopedic surgery; Joanie Huggins who kept me clothed, fed and sane during this lengthy project.

Library of Congress Cataloging in Publication Data

Huggins, Hal A
Why raise ugly kids?

Bibliography: p.
Includes index.
1. Children—Care and hygiene. 2. Children—Nutrition. 3. Beauty, Personal. 4. Abnormalities, Human—Etiology. 5. Children—Sleep. 6. Sleep positions. I. Title.
RJ61.H893 1981 613'.0432 80-28733
ISBN 0-87000-507-3

MANUFACTURED IN THE UNITED STATES OF AMERICA

0 9 8 7 6 5 4 3 2 1

To the memory of one of earth's most creative minds. May we always remember that Dr. Harvey Stallard made earth a better place to live.

Contents

Foreword

This is a bright, cheerful, helpful, hopeful book. Dr. Huggins has a unique facility for dropping clues all along the trail and then letting the curious reader put together his "own" conclusions.

He makes frequent reference to Dr. Weston Price, whose book *Nutrition and Physical Degeneration* should be required reading for every sixth grader. Because of his respect for this late, great dentist, I am trapped into believing everything—well, almost everything—that Dr. Huggins says.

He points the way for the reader to make correct connections in a very readable, conversational style. Softer facial bones *will* get pushed around if a child is a prone sleeper. We should make an effort to get babies to sleep on their backs. Many cow's-milk-fed babies have colic; maybe they are not absorbing the milk stolen from the calf. If they were breast fed, they would be less likely to have colic, be more likely to absorb calcium better, and have better dental arches (because the strong lips of the breast-fed baby keep the teeth in line). "Ugly" pinched faces and droopy shoulders may be brought on by diet and sleeping position. Such "ugliness" is probably multifactoral, but I appreciate the fact that Dr. Huggins points out a new option.

I agree with Dr. Huggins that hyperactive children are trying to signal us that they do not feel good. Magnesium is usually low in these children. I have found that calcium is usually low also. Milk—at least homogenized-pasturized milk—may be the villain, as absorption of calcium from it is faulty and it contains no magnesium.

For a number of reasons, I'm not sure that I can share Dr. Huggins' enthusiasm for honey, but the stuff is useful in weaning a "sugarholic" off the really bad refined carbohydrates. Sweet-tasting foods other than fruits and breast milk just promote the idea that everything must taste sweet; that food philosophy must cease. Joanie Huggins' tips are valuable aids in helping us all, child and adult alike, get off the junk.

Thank you, Dr. Huggins, for giving insights and opening our eyes to new ways of looking at old problems. Keep questioning the old ways. Help us seek ultimate truth, even it if hurts.

May I eat one eclair a year?*

LENDON SMITH, MD

* Yes, Lendon, as long as I get my yearly Ghirardelli hot fudge sundae.—H.A.H.

Do I Want to Read This Book?

Here's what it's all about . . .

Why Raise Ugly Kids? is an all-encompassing title. Our first reaction is to think of ugly faces and bodies. But what about other uglies? The hyperkinetic child is ugly. The child who claws at discipline due to a lack of self-esteem is ugly. Whether we are Miss Americas or Miss Celaneouses, we lose our beauty after three days in bed with a cold. If our teeth are full of holes or our faces full of pimples, we shun the mirror. If kids can't relate to why their parents want them to eat "stuff that's good for us," they can get pretty ugly.

I don't know of a better way to describe any of these scenes than Ugly. Why be ugly when with a little direction we could be beautiful?

After spending ten years doing the studies that Dr. Harvey Stallard suggested, I'm convinced that most of our ugliness is self-inflicted. A lot of ugliness wouldn't happen if we didn't make it happen. That's what this book is all about—finding out how to avoid forcing Mother Nature to go wrong and produce Ugly Kids, keeping Mother Nature from going wrong.

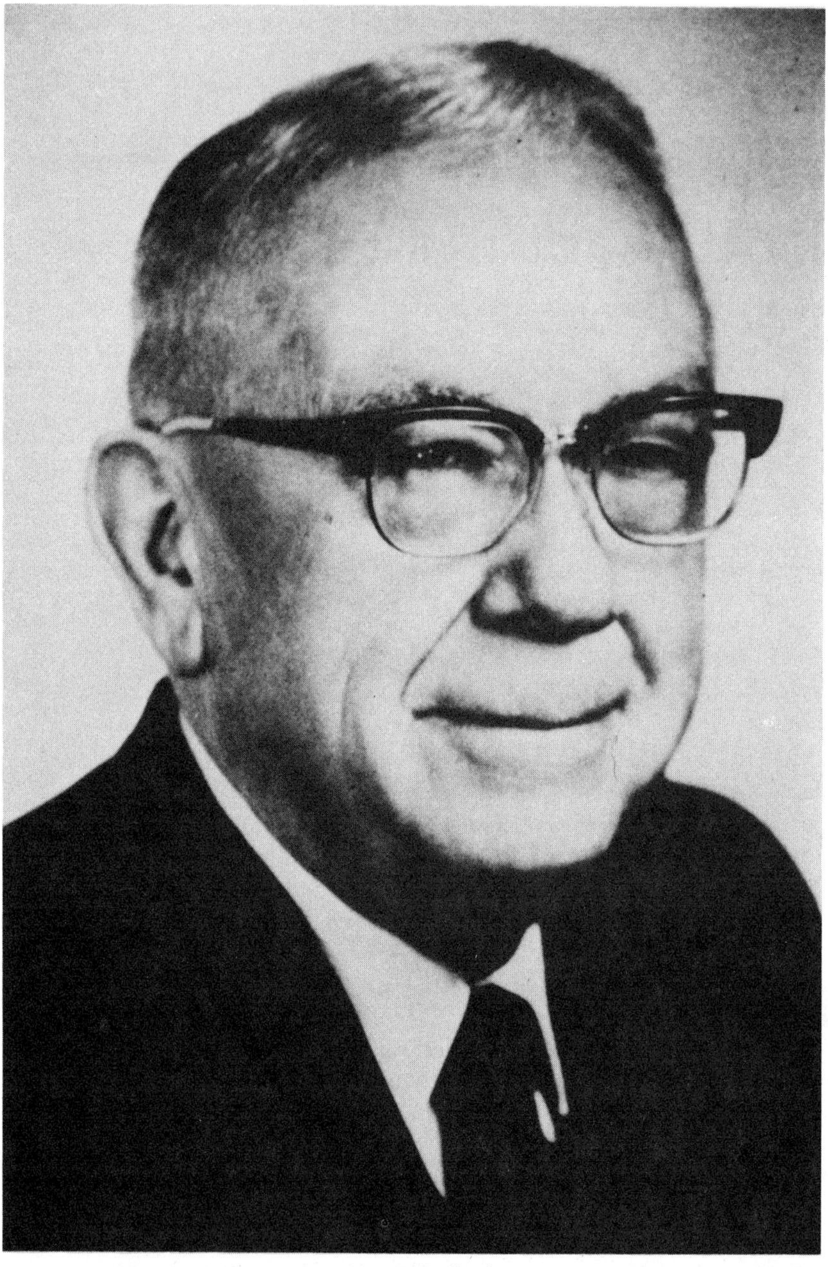

Harvey Stallard

Tribute to Harvey Stallard

Harvey Stallard grew up close to the soil. He was raised on a Kansas farm with an appreciation for rebuilding soils after reaping a harvest. He recognized then that healthy bodies are related to healthy plants and soils.

Dinnertime set the stage for his lifestyle at meals by his father's leading the family in discussions of Shakespeare, Tennyson, Whitman, current events, and classical literature. Farming and other daily problems were never mentioned at mealtime.

Obviously he was well read, though he refused to let literature bind him. After receiving his first doctorate in education and agriculture (1909), he taught for several years. He had his own methods of education. "You learn best by doing, and, oppositely, you learn less by reading books, and you learn to think less if you depend upon authorities."

He earned his second doctorate in botany in 1917. Because of his involvement in civil service he found himself, during the First World War, directing dental activities. Dentistry looked interesting, so he obtained his third doctorate in dentistry in 1920. He was interested in orthodontics, so felt that he slighted such subjects as surgery. Slight it or not, his surgery notes were uesd as a syllabus by future students for years. He then went on to further studies for proficiency in orthodontics.

By the mid-1920s Harvey began to wonder about those 52 tooth buds folded into a skull of more than 40 bones. He undertook to study children and their sleeping habits and to publish the results of his findings.

Sleeping on the face, he maintained, during a child's early formative years could produce malposed tooth buds. His ideas met with a complacent, mundane reception. He continued his research and observations for more than ten years before putting them aside. He was to wait until nearly 1970 before a young dentist came to sit at his feet and develop a consuming interest in pursuing his observations on sleeping habits.

Why Raise Ugly Kids?

Why Raise Ugly Kids?

We are but tenants of our skin, no one can thus deny
The one who made and holds the lease lives way up in the sky.
We give our body care and food to nurture as our goal
And as a just and fair reward we get to keep our soul.

But should we fail to do our part, the upkeep and the rent,
The landlord has his time of grace, then out of shape gets bent.
Or should you harm or lay to waste the body you call home
The landlord's notice will be served, you'll find yourself alone.

That great white horse will haunt your door, he'll find you gaunt
and tired,
And tell you five immortal words, "Your lease has now expired."

You've lost the right to drive the cart, that's why I sent the horse.
Your friends will cry and call it death, but you will know remorse.

So while you're young and growing strong and taking hold the reins,
Take care to watch of what you eat, what runs within your veins,
Learn what to do to pull you through, and when to ply the skids,
Cause no one wants the lousy task of raising Ugly Kids.

Chapter One

Why Raise Ugly Teeth?

A revolutionary new concept: Crooked teeth are not inherited. We (frequently as parents) do something that makes them crooked.

My whole outlook toward the human race changed as a result of Dr. Harvey Stallard's challenge to me a few years ago. I now understand why he had such an impact on dentistry during his 63 years of practice. He had a unique ability to jar men off dead center and send them rolling posthaste in the direction best suited for their abilities. In my case it was toward sleep.

When I look at people today my eyes wander to the position of shoulder blades, the curves in their spines, the position of their feet, crooked noses, crooked teeth and receding chins. I do this because I know that all of these characteristics can be influenced by the way people sleep. The study of sleeping positions was my first introduction to the realization that people are not *born* pretty or ugly, but often what we as parents do to them can influence the way their faces look. The study of sleeping habits was a lesson in "how the twig is bent," for there are forces at work on facial bones while we sleep. As the pressure is applied, so the bone grows.

I had heard Dr. Harvey Stallard's name mentioned once during a discussion of the origins of orthodontic problems. Several people laughed.

"What's so funny?" I asked.

"Harvey wouldn't agree with that—he thinks sleeping habits cause crooked teeth."

"Sleeping habits?" The words stuck. They kept bounding back and forth between my conscious and subconscious mind. It was as if a book full of blank pages sat in my subconscious. It kept asking me to put words on the pages. I finally called Dr. Stallard and asked if I could visit him. I didn't know why for sure. I just knew I had to go.

Shortly after I arrived at his office, Dr. Stallard and I were talking—well, he was talking and I was listening—about research he and a group of pediatricians had done with the staff of the San Diego City and County Health Department during the 1920s. The study involved recording changes in growth and development in children during an eight-year period. They examined 6,772 children of various racial backgrounds aged birth to 17 years. At the end of their eight-year study, the doctors were quoted as saying, "Most babies at birth have a few faults in forms, but after 12 months many have serious faults." There was a hidden clue within that sentence, as well as in the one Stallard published for dentists: "Most of these babies at birth appeared to have faces free of faults, but after 12 months many had serious faults in their faces."

Of keen interest to Harvey Stallard were the changes that occurred during the first *two* years of life. He had found that 98 percent of the children had normal facial development at birth and 2 percent had "congenital malformations." Research rules dictated that the children be retested at ages 3, 6, 12, and 24 months. Stallard found that the three-month study essentially duplicated the birth figures, but surprisingly, by age 24 months the percentage of improper facial development had jumped from 2 to 50. These figures reflect the number of children who will some day require orthodontic treatment. That was a fantastic increase for such a short period of time. By age 17 these percentages had climbed from 50 percent to 68 percent—but this was an increase of only 36 percent during the 15-year span from age two to 17 as compared to a 2,400 percent increase from birth to age two years. To summarize, Stallard found:

Birth	2%	Congenital facial malformation
3 months	2%	Facial malformation
2 years	50%	Facial malformation
17 years	68%	Facial malformation

After these studies were completed, Stallard began to question the age-old memorized answers to the question of why kids have crooked teeth. Up to that time (and even today) many dentists thought that crooked teeth were the result of heredity or poor dental treatment during a child's early years. None of the old answers made sense when examined in the light of this new evidence.

The most popular story among the old answers was the "melting pot" theory. Hometown girls married hometown boys centuries ago. This was part tradition and part lack of telephones and automobiles. In America (the "melting pot") ancestral heritage is not well defined—we are all "Americans." Most of us have practiced a form of what might be called *European intermarriage.* If your father was a big Polish man, and your mother a tiny French gal, couldn't you inherit his big Polish teeth and her little French jaw? That makes sense when you think of someone in your family who has daddy's eye color and mother's hair color. Sure it could happen. Many parents and doctors have been quite satisfied with this explanation.

Another popular explanation I used to use is the "hardness of the diet" story. Children of bygone centuries ate raw meat and tough food. It is reported that they chewed with a force of 500 pounds per square inch. We know that if one exercises a muscle extensively it will develop to maximum size. Wow! Of course. Look at Charles Atlas! Remember the pictures on the back pages of the comic books? The 97-pound weakling? He was on the beach when a ruffian kicked sand on his girlfriend, and in telling off the big fellow our 97-pounder came in second best. Humiliation in front of his girlfriend. Trauma! All he did was to work out on some Charles Atlas exercise springs and in the next picture he had developed a Mr. America body. He then proceeded to punch the sand-kicking fellow in the nose. From stories like this, our minds can easily relate exercise to body development. This makes the chewing-hard-food story sound scientific.

A candidate for third place that *really* makes sense is the "premature-loss-of-teeth" story. Any dentist who has removed an abscessed baby tooth years before it would normally be lost has had the opportunity to see the tooth behind it drift *forward.*

Another "cause" of crooked teeth is the tonsil and adenoid problem. When the nose becomes more or less permanently clogged due to infection and swelling of the tonsils and adenoids this causes "perverted mechanics." This means a change in breathing habits using the mouth instead of the nose to breathe through. This is supposed to create a type of air passage which slows down development of the lower jaw enough to produce a gearlike fit of upper teeth to lower teeth. The resulting smaller lower jaw changes the direction of force applied to the teeth during chewing and directs forces backward in the base of the lower jaw, thus preventing its forward growth.

This is an extremely complicated explanation, but it was satisfying to the academic mind of a few decades ago, and as with many things in science, since it had been quoted a lot, it *must* be true. Almost anyone can relate to tonsil and adenoid problems, so this theory stood for some years, awaiting the piercing eye of Harvey Stallard.

Occasionally the *upper* jaw is underdeveloped. Atmospheric pressure has been blamed for this defect. The small upper jaw is said to be due to the small upper lip and negative atmospheric pressure within the nose (which occurs inhaling). This permits the relatively higher air pressure next to the cheek to exert pressure against the cheeks and nose leading to a collapse of the upper jaw. In other words, as we inhale, we create a partial vacuum within our noses that allows the surrounding air to mash in our faces. On this basis, what do you suppose a *sneeze* does? This negative pressure from inhaling also results in pulling the palate (roof of the mouth) upward, producing a high, narrow palate and, at the same time, pushing the nasal septum (the middle bone dividing the nostrils) to one side. This is called the deviated septum. Obviously the "deviated" septum and "perverted" masticatory forces were named a generation gap ago. We have a few chapters to go before we are introduced to the deviated swallow and its friends, but rest assured that none of these subjects have anything to do with sex. They are merely technical words that have wandered around a generation or two looking for a place in the popular vocabulary.

Thumb-sucking is an explanation for crooked teeth that dates back over a century. Obviously, something as large as a thumb occupies space that would normally be held by teeth, so its presence would conceivably distort bones and move teeth. A runner-up to the thumb theory is the bottle-feeding theory. Baby bottles have been blamed for types of malocclusion similar to those produced by the thumb. The bottle is given two counts, though, one mechanical, by providing pressure, and the second, chemical, because the contents are not considered adequate to duplicate normal nutrition found in mother's milk.

The tongue resides in the mouth and is a muscle of near constant motion. If misdirected in its activities, surely the strong tongue muscle could move teeth out of position. Some children have been known to habitually bite their tongues. Others "thrust" it during swallowing. There are even cases of overgrowth, producing an abnormally large tongue.

Stallard looked over all of this in light of the observations he had made on almost 7,000 children, and he was not able to accept the "usual explanations" anymore. In researching the literature he found only two cases that suggested what he termed *extraoral pressures* as a cause of malocclusion. One article, by Dr. George Baker, had appeared in 1903, and the other, by Dr. Calvin Case, was written about 1918. It seemed that Stallard had stumbled onto something that had the potential to uproot a century of thinking.

* * *

"Know anything about farming?" Harvey asked me one afternoon in his laboratory. I was looking over orthodontic plaster casts of gross-looking crooked teeth.

"Well, both my grandfathers had farms," I replied.

"Know anything about experimental embryology?" he asked next.

"Yes," I replied. "My roommate in college worked in the biology department one summer and did some animal experiments at that time."

"Pretty modern stuff, eh?"

"Yes, lots of sophisticated equipment."

"Learn a lot?"

"I suppose so."

"New field, this experimental embryology."

I should have known he was setting me up. Harvey seldom got into conversations by accident. He was always trying to encourage people to be observant. His favorite trick was to show a young man that he had seen many things but observed little. I always had the feeling that Harvey was wearing magnifying lenses while the rest of us were wearing dark glasses.

"I used to do experimental embryology," said Harvey.

"Oh, when?" I knew he had BS, PhD, PhB, DSc, and DDS degrees, but when did he have time to do experimental embryology?

"'Round the turn of the century."

"You did experimental embryology in 1900?" I exclaimed, aghast. "That's a *new* field. How did you know anything about it then?"

"*Everyone* did then. In Kansas. You know what a mule is, don't you?"

"Yes, it's an animal born of a cross between two other animals that can't reproduce itself."

"Know what two animals?"

"Horse and something."

"Horse and donkey. Cross them and you get a fine work animal. Used them a lot on the farm. Had some real nice ones at one time." Then he paused for awhile.

"Know what? Never saw a mule with a horse's teeth and a donkey's jaw."

Zing! I had been zinged. Experimental biology. In the laboratory all kinds of bugs were being crossed with other bugs to see what would happen. That was experimental embryology to me. Here on a big scale Harvey had just exploded one of my prize explanations of where crooked teeth came from.

"But those are animals."

Harvey just looked at me with no expression. I got the idea that some questions were worthy of conversation and others were too obvious to merit consideration.

"Know how many kids have crooked teeth?"

"Lots."

"Nearly three-fourths. Maybe more now. More coming on all the time."

"Guess it's always been that way."

"Trouble with young folks. No perspective. See something for ten years and start talking about 'always.' I've driven a team of horses more miles than you've walked—yes, I've seen men walk on the moon too. Lot's happened in between. You know, young folks ought to study history more. See how things change. Just because it's now doesn't mean it's always been."

"You trying to tell me crooked teeth are something new?"

"Not only new, but isolated. You know there are places *today* where *no one* has crooked teeth?"

"On earth?"

"Yep. Amazon valley. Leastwise up through the fifties. Don't know for sure about now. May be infested with white men now."

"Interracial marriage?"

"Nope. Thoughts. Everywhere Americans go they infect people with their way of thinking. Look at the Eskimos. Perfectly healthy people 'till we influenced them."

"You've lost me. First Amazons and straight teeth, now Eskimos and poor health. What's the connection?"

"Maybe you didn't know," he said, "crooked teeth are a disease—a degenerative disease, or in line with your recently trained college mind—a metabolic disorder."

"Disease?" My mind sank. My conscious ability to wrestle with words submerged into the oblivion of confusion known as stupor. It's a time when the expression on one's face relieves him of the responsibility of fending for himself.

"You've had enough for one day," I remember hearing Harvey say. "I'll call you a cab and we can meet here at my office about 7:30 in the morning."

I can't be sure of what I did that evening—probably stared at a wall. Disease? My dental training flashed before me that night along with Harvey's pearls of wisdom dropped during the day. I knew I would have to think or swim. Either I would open my mind like a big window and let the new rays of knowledge take over or pack up and go home secure in documented publications. I slept.

* * *

"Well, how do you feel this morning?" asked Harvey. He was already fooling around in the laboratory at 7:30 A.M., and, from the looks of the floor, had been doing so for some time. Dentists are notoriously sloppy with plaster, orthodontists or not.

"Dumb," I replied, "I feel dumb."

He stopped mixing plaster and looked at me. I felt he was looking at my soul.

"You're ready to learn aren't you, son?"

"Yes," I said, sounding as impassioned as I could. Then I felt a tear slip out of my left eye and run down my cheek. He spotted it. I turned away and picked up a cast. I don't know where that tear came from, but I felt my face flush. I was embarrassed. I felt pressure in my ears, then it moved forward and pushed out two more tears. What was happening to me? Harvey knew.

"You know, young man," he said from across the room. "I think you're going to take this sleeping habits thing and make something out of it. In fact, I think I'll live another two or three years just to see if you can." With that he opened the door to his private office and I stepped into a new world. I knew I was committed.

* * *

What about heredity? Doesn't that have some role in facial development? Harvey looked upon heredity as a gas tank. Simply put, if an airplane gets one mile to the gallon and you are going 100 miles, would you start with 100 gallons? Not if you want to arrive in one piece. A one-mile-an-hour head wind would render you short of the mark. Heredity is our potential. Only this and nothing more. I don't *really* think we can exceed it, but there are many things we can do to create head winds or cross winds in our heredity development journey. Anything in the line of poor diet, deficiencies, sickness or habits can keep us from attaining the full measure of our individual potential.

Harvey's suggestions led me to read the work of Weston Price, DDS. Dr. Price traveled the world extensively during the 1930s. He found many areas of the world where people were relatively free from orthodontic problems. He wrote of studying skulls—as many as 8,000 in one area—and finding one cavity per 1,000 teeth. Orthodontic problems were about as rare. Maybe Stallard was right. Perhaps crooked teeth are a recent development in humans.

Stallard told me of people he knew living in San Diego who had some children born in Europe and some born in the United States. Line them up in a row, and there was an obvious difference in appearance. Anyone could divide them into two groups, but it took Stallard to tell *why* they looked different. Did the parents change their heredity by crossing the Atlantic? Some anthropologists I have spoken with mention promiscuity as the reason. No, I don't think so, not after looking at the large numbers of pictures that Price took. He could show the same differences that Stallard was talking about in families that stayed in the same area. It was Weston Price who emphasized even more than Stallard that biochemical disturbances in growth produce crooked teeth. I was led to find that every one of the leaning habits, sleeping positions, and nutritional insults that Stallard kept expounding on contributed its part to faulty facial development, and it was clear that *all* these areas had to be investigated to see how much each contributed to crooked teeth and narrow faces. No *one* part was going to be the total key to raising nice-looking kids free from facial faults.

Harvey's early publications led to criticism from geneticists who argued about facial similarities in families. Harvey's point was that if the parents slept all their kids the same way, the kids would all look alike. He was referring to narrow faces, depressed cheek bones, crowded teeth and small chins. As the twig is bent, so grows the tree. Harvey's point was that genetics rarely gives us deformed faces—only 2 percent of the time. He kept making the point that a *lack* of heredity force produced deformed faces.

Dr. Weston Price's work also showed facial similarities—not only in families but in races of people. He found an amazing number of similarities among facial structures until the white man's diet was introduced to the child-bearing women and young children. Dr. Price used figure 1 to show racial facial similarities in nonrelated boys living on separate islands. They look as if they could be brothers, but their only relationship is racial. Their ancestors were probably of the same tribe hundreds of generations ago, and the facial characteristics have been preserved through the years by giving each generation adequate heredity force with a minimum of interference.

Harvey Stallard emphasized Price's work and added his own observation that specific abnormalities in facial development were associated with specific abnormal pressures during sleep in over 7,000 cases. It was

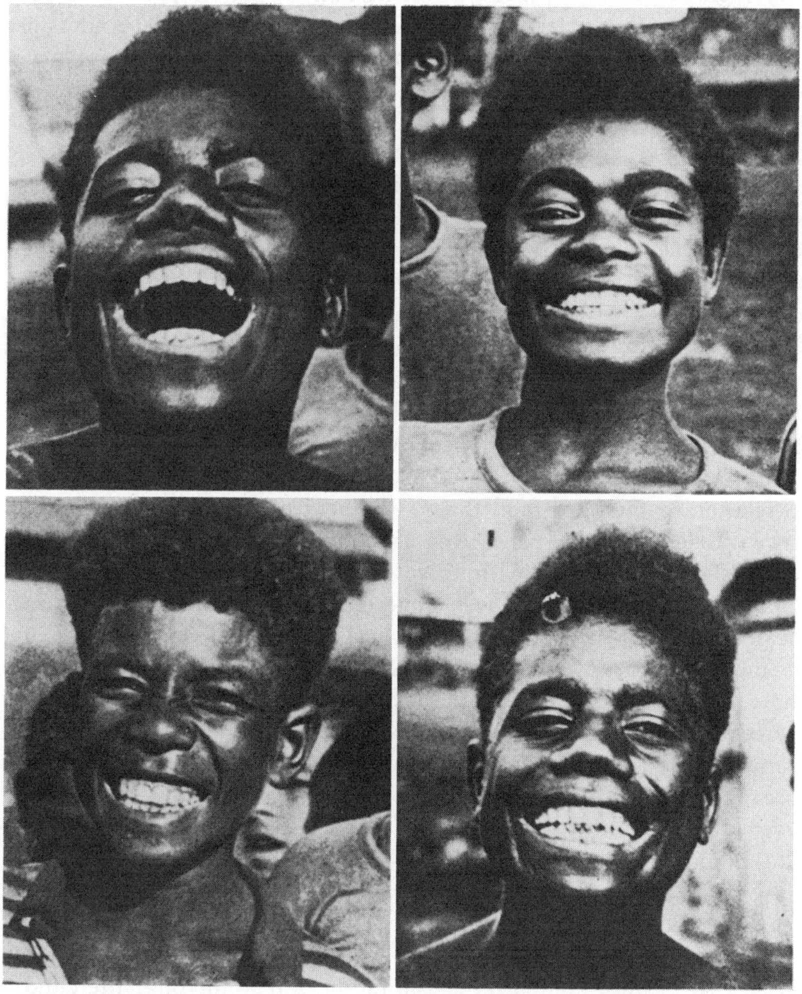

Figure 1

logical to associate cause and effect. The simplicity of his concept was its biggest enemy.

* * *

Hardness of the diet—I can remember this being discussed in school. A man named Lamarck once expressed the theory that "exercise of the special function of an organ is necessary for its full volumetric development." It was felt that the Indians of America and especially the primitive and ancient peoples ate foods far less refined than ours, therefore they exercised more muscular effort in eating than we do. It has been suggested that the ancient peoples chewed with a force of 500 pounds per square inch compared with our 20 pounds of force in eating an apple pie. This would explain *their* full facial development and *lack* of crooked teeth. That sounded logical enough, but Stallard suggested *searching it out.*

"Read about ancient diets and child cultures."

Reading about the foods available to ancient Greeks and Romans, I found the following to be available: grapes, apples, pomegranates, melons, dates, figs, milk, eggs, honey, cheese, mushrooms, asparagus, artichokes, oysters, fish, game, goat, mutton and wheat bread. That doesn't sound dramatically different from what is available today, and certainly wouldn't require excessive muscular development to chew. With so much emphasis placed on hardness of diet, I felt surprise at finding a menu so nonsupportive of the theory.

Indian and Eskimo diets looked as if they were going to show a closer correlation to the hard-food theory. Both races ate lots of meat (raw, jerky, broiled or stewed) and often used their hands and teeth to tear the food instead of cutting it with knives and forks. Of course, raw meat is not usually tough—in fact, well-done meat is harder to chew than raw meat. Perhaps the preparation and consistency is not so different, just the method of cutting it up. Cornmeal was an Indian staple, but records show that it was ground to about the consistency we find in crackers.

Keeping in mind that the majority of the malformations Stallard had found occurred *before* the age of two years, I studied "uncivilized" cultures, as well as Indian and Eskimo. I found that most of these children were breast-fed until *after* the age of two. Now if a child of *any* culture bites mother's breast with 500 pounds of force . . .

In many ancient cultures, as a child developed a few teeth and his needs for food exceeded what mother's milk could supply, the mother would chew the food first, then place it in the child's mouth. Gross! This doesn't fit modern standards of sanitation, but it *did* offer the child a method of getting *Lactobacillus acidophilus. Lactobacillus* is a digestion-abiding bug that helps prevent cholic and other stomach disorders. How *Lactobacillus* can improve carbohydrate digestion will be discussed more thoroughly later.

According to Professor Blumni in *Home Life of Ancient Greeks,* children were breast-fed by either the mother or a wet nurse as long as three years. Either the mother or the nurse chewed harder food until the child had its baby molars.

* * *

What about the premature-loss-of-baby-teeth theory? One of the first things I was taught in the department of pedodontics (dentistry for children) was how to make a space maintainer. A space maintainer is a dental appliance usually attached to one or more teeth next to where a baby tooth was prematurely lost. A wire spanning the vacant space keeps the remaining teeth from moving into that space. If a child's tooth had to be removed before the permanent tooth was ready to erupt, we placed space maintainers within a week or so. Stallard was also a proponent of this theory until he looked at the results of his study. He still placed space maintainers. So do I, but not with the feeling of pride in having prevented an orthodontic problem that I used to have.

In studying children in the San Diego area, Stallard found many ethnic groups. At that time (the 1920s) ethnic groups in America tended to practice many traditions from their homeland. (This is not seen so much today. People from other countries tend to adopt the American culture faster than they did in the early 1900s.) It became evident that two extremes existed in San Diego: those who got a lot of dental care and those who got practically none. The Caucasian kids received the most "six-month recalls," which included cleaning and X-raying the teeth. Cavities were filled in baby teeth and space maintainers were used frequently. Japanese children got practically none of these services. When a tooth hurt badly enough, Harvey told me, the father would take hold with a pair of pliers and remove it in his own fashion. This home-craft surgery was sometimes the total dental service that a Japanese child in San Diego knew in the 1920s.

There was also one other great divider of ethnic groups. Who had the most cases of crooked teeth and who had the least? First place—that is, the *most* cases of crooked teeth—went to Caucasians. Wouldn't you know it—the *least* number of cases per population was found in the Japanese. How do the facts sit with the dental ego? Not well at all!

Looking at the total figures from Stallard's study, Japanese children had the *highest* number of decayed teeth, the *most* abscessed teeth and the *earliest* loss of baby teeth—but the *least* number of crooked teeth. Looking at these facts surely did change my thinking on the subject of what *really* causes crooked teeth. In attempting to show which type of malocclusion (dental lingo for *crooked teeth*) was most related to early tooth loss, Stallard found practically *no* connection between tooth loss and malocclusion. He finally listed early-tooth-loss as a "negligible causal factor." Probably the most fatal comment in regard to the early-tooth-loss theory was the discovery that nearly every classification of crooked teeth appeared in children's mouths who had *not lost any* teeth prematurely.

Stallard finally concluded that dentists did *not* cause malocclusion by failing to fill decayed baby teeth *or* by neglecting to place space maintainers. There was something more going on. Somehow dentists had the idea that tooth growth controlled jaw growth. Maybe the problem was of greater magnitude than that. What Harvey had noted in his child studies was more than displaced teeth. He had written of mismated jaws, where the bony size of one jaw did not match the size of the other, misshapen faces—narrow jaws that provided an environment excellent for producing crowded teeth, and something else that's ugly, impacted wisdom teeth. He had noted that the sunken-in cheekbones produced a saddened expression in the happiest of children's faces. Surely these things were the result of more than the premature loss of a tooth.

* * *

Stallard had a challenge for the theory of tonsilitis and inflamed adenoids being the cause of crooked teeth. These problems were attributed to such environmental factors at house confinement, improper clothing, and a race congested in dense populations which made epidemics possible. Advocates of this theory prescribed exercises for the jaws, throat, lips and chest to overcome the "perverted respiration" that resulted from nasal congestion.

This theory could not account for *one* major problem: the vast majority of orthodontic problems are *unilateral*. That is, they are far more severe on *one* side than on the other. If air pressure is going to affect a bone it has to do it equally, like blowing up a balloon. Equal pressures should produce equal malformations. How could air pressure be selective to just one side of the face?

Thumb-sucking obviously presents a hazard to proper development.

This in itself is variable because some thumb suckers have gross deformities while others show only slight or no evidence of the habit. This is due to several reasonably obvious facts; it depends upon how much sucking pressure is applied, how much jaw muscle pressure is used, and how much time is spent practicing the habit. One interesting fact that Stallard found is that, during a period of sickness, frequently the facial bones are more plastic, that is, they are softer and can be molded easier. That means that if a child has a prolonged illness and indulges in a thumb- or finger-sucking habit, it will do *greater* harm than the same length of time and intensity of sucking in a healthy child.

Bottle feeding has long been known to be responsible for the formation of loose, flaccid lips, as shown in figure 2. *Prickard's bottle mouth* is the term applied to lips shaped like this. They have little muscle tone and are frequently too flaccid to provide the balance for tongue pressure. Teeth come and settle where they are due to a balance between two opposite muscle forces—those of the lips and the tongue. There is a little horseshoe-shaped area of equilibrium between these two forces, and that's

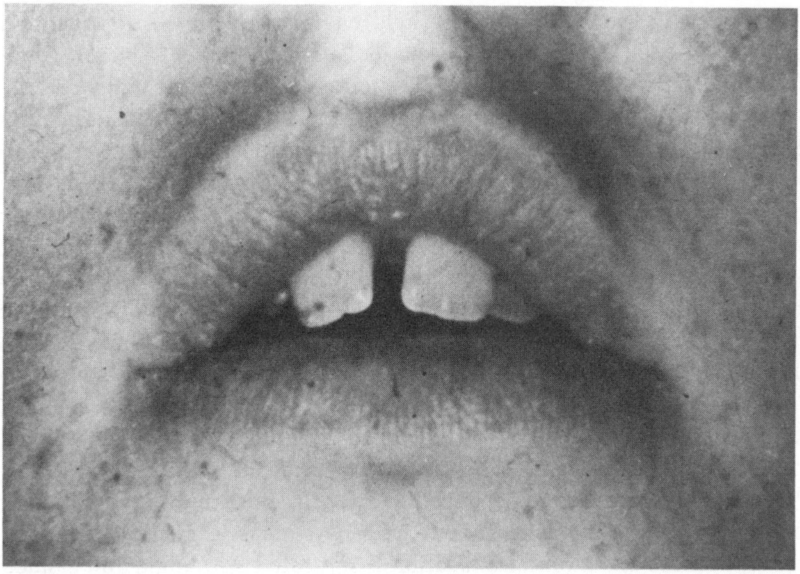

Figure 2

where the teeth rest. If the lips are weak and the tongue is strong, then the front teeth move forward. This can cause space between the teeth or can cause the "Bucky Beaver" appearance. If the tongue rests *between* the teeth, a condition known as the *open* bite results. This means that the front teeth don't touch even when the back teeth are together. There are two basic types of crooked teeth covered by the term *open bite.* One is when the upper and lower teeth are headed for each other in closing, but the back teeth hit before the front ones get close to each other. The other (far more serious) is when the whole upper bony arch is pushed forward. I have seen cases of this so severe that the kid could not touch his front teeth together even when sticking his chin forward as far as he could.

The number two problem with bottle feeding deserves a lot of discussion—and will get it. Proteins, vitamins, minerals, hormones, sugars and antibodies are usually supplied in the proper amounts in mother's milk. No artificial milk-substitute has yet been invented to rival the quality, cost, or convenience of nature's own.

* * *

Last year Joanie (my wife) and I took David and Kathy (our kids) on a two-day raft trip down the Colorado River. I remember our apprehension as we approached the first rapids on our six-man rubber raft. First we heard the rushing sounds of tumbling water. Then we heard the roar. Then we saw it. Spellbound, we held on for dear life as the boatman skillfully guided us into what looked like a roller coaster of water. Mom was the first to scream. Her hat flew off. She lunged for it toward the center of the raft just as we dropped our first three feet. This was just enough to throw her off balance and she went down on her hands and knees into a torrent of rushing water that nearly engulfed the raft. Fear of the unknown was justified. Another drop—another tidal wave of water over our heads—now we were *all* screaming and hanging onto the raft with all our strength. Just as we were getting really wet and used to the tumble action, all was calm. The rapids were over. Still water. We looked around and it was obvious who got the worst dunking. Mom. There she was—in the bottom of the boat, still on all fours—soaked to the skin. Her blond hair looked like Phyllis Diller's on a bad day, but of all things, she was smiling. As she regained what was left of her soaked composure, she grinned real big and said, "How far to the next rapids?"

This is how Stallard left me feeling after tossing me into the rapids of his thoughts. I was dashed about with new ideas, flailed by recurring thoughts from my "formal education," saturated with logic and calmed by the evidence Harvey was showing me in his patients' mouths. How far to the next rapids? I knew there was no turning back. As someone once said, "A mind once stretched by a new idea will never return to its original shape." Stallard had stretched my mind far enough to accept new concepts of facial development, but somehow I felt that this was just the beginning.

Chapter Two

Why Cause Poor Postures?

Stooped shoulders, just like crooked teeth, are caused, not inherited. Mother, stop telling Johnnie to stand up straight if you are the one who gave him poor posture. Help him to correct it permanently.

"Packaging!" Stallard looked up from a patient into what I feel was my blankest expression. "Packaging, that's the secret."

This was the first English sentence he had said in half an hour. As teenage patients came in Harvey would ask what language they were studying. After finding out, he would spend the entire appointment speaking in that language. I was in a blissful, noncoherent state of smiling pleasantly to the sound of French when he had broken the spell by saying, "Packaging." I was ready to hand him an instrument and was not really prepared for the *challenge* he was so famous for issuing.

"If you could design a modern method of packaging children then you would cut down the incidence of crooked teeth to a fraction of what it is now. Nutrition—follow-up with that and you'd have a real *'package deal.'* " He chuckled to himself over this pun and returned to a French discussion of how to keep braces cleaner. With a shrug to me the patient popped out of the chair and said, "They don't teach you that sort of stuff in school. Only verbs."

As the patient left I remarked, "How many languages do you speak?"

"Oh, I don't know—depends on what's needed."

"Needed?"

"Yes, as the need arises. Once I was asked to speak in Portugal. Now those poor souls don't have command of the English technical vocabulary enough to understand a discussion of intricate movements of the jaw presented in gnathology, so I took six weeks to learn *their* language. It would have been an insult to them for me to be their guest and then have me speak to them in a foreign language, wouldn't it?"

"They have interpreters."

"Oh, yes, and they do fine with 'I'm so glad to be here' and 'It was a lovely dinner,' but I had to discuss a technical viewpoint with them and I wanted to be sure they understood me. You'd do the same thing, wouldn't you?"

Confronted with the monumental task of learning a language in six weeks, I decided to change the subject before I was "challenged" again.

"What would I talk about—sleeping habits?" I asked in a diversionary manner. It worked.

"Oh, yes, that. . ." Good. His mind was back to the present monumental task.

"Now, tell you what you can do." He hesitated a moment and looked me squarely in the eyes as if he had forgotten something.

"You live in Colorado, don't you?"

"Yes."

"That's not far from New Mexico and Arizona. Call Goldwater, tell him what you are interested in and ask his advice. He wrote a book on Indians—has a lot of honest interest. Tell him I sent you."

"Barry Goldwater? The Senator?"

"Yes."

"You know him?"

"Know lots of political people. We need them. They need us. That's how things get done. Cleveland told me that once."

"Grover Cleveland? That's a long time ago."

"Not too long—I've worked with every president since Woodrow Wilson. Worked with him when San Diego was just a pup of a town. We designed the sewage disposal system at that time. Still using basically the same ideas. Helped lay out the streets, too. He was a good man. Liked working with him. Liked Ike too. Now there's a back sleeper for you, Ike. Good posture, fine figure of a man—told him so, too. Anyway, get down into New Mexico and Arizona. Go to the Amazon. With air travel today it wouldn't take any time at all. Don't go to Alaska—too Americanized—read about it in Price's book, *Nutrition and Physical Degeneration.*"

He continued discussing my project and pointed out the importance of a multidisciplined approach. "Check with orthopedic surgeons, osteopaths, psychiatrists. Read, go, look, *see.* That's the important thing—don't just look, but *see.* Study opposing views, draw conclusions, challenge them . . .

"Harvey?"

He seemed surprised to have me interrupt his 90-mile-an-hour checklist. He stopped in his tracks like a television instant replay, fully intending to carry on at the same speed after I had asked my question.

"What am I doing anyway? I seem to have gotten lost somewhere between Arizona and the Amazon."

"Package, boy, package."

"Kids?"

"Of course. That's their trouble. We *let* them get into trouble. Even force it on 'em. Got to stop doing that. That's your job. Teach people how to package their kids."

Package—now it began to fit. Forces—we have to control the forces. "Harvey—what's the first part of the head to calcify?"

He leaned back, looked at me with a big grin on his face, and said, "Now you're thinking. That's what you went to school for. Review your anatomy. Why, back of the head, of course. Occiput. Starts the day of birth. Sort of makes sense to put the weight there, doesn't it? What about the front of the head? Remember that?"

No I didn't, so I just looked at him expectantly.

"Two years. Kids are two years old before those thin membrane bones begin to calcify. By then it's too late for most of them, but you can sure help *anytime* before they're seventeen. Helps afterward too, though, 'cause pressure on the face keeps moving teeth all your life."

I decided I had better pin Harvey down to the basics before he had me too deep into other projects to remember why he had started me on this one. Where did it all start? Harvey doesn't really start, he just begins. Starting implies that there is a step one somewhere. I guessed I'd have to find that later.

There was the restaurant. That's the place where he really blew my mind. One morning I was watching him practice orthodontics when he looked up at me and inquired as to my feelings about ethnic foods.

"I really like them." I replied. "East Indian is my favorite, but I really like Mexican food." This seemed logical enough to me, because San Diego is close to Tiajuana, and I assumed he was indirectly asking me if I like Mexican food. "I don't eat it Sunday evening through Friday noon, of course."

"Why not?"

He was baiting me. I didn't know it. I thought I had best educate him though.

"Mexican food stays on your breath—you know—the onion and garlic. Well, if I ate that during the week, I wouldn't have to use novocaine on my patients. Just exhale."

He seemed to miss the humor. "You can't get rid of the odor?"

"Nope. It can't be done."

"Trouble with young folks."

"Trouble?"

"You don't look—just take old folks' word for everything."

"Well I. . ."

Later I found out that no one really gets very far trying to outguess Harvey. I eventually learned to just smile and mentally brace myself for another set of rapids.

"I like Mexican food—hotter the better," he said. "Sneak off to Tiajuana twice a week to a little hole in the wall that really puts out pure ethnic meals. Most Mexicans can't take it as hot as I can. Folks here at the office think I take a nap. I have to keep it mum. They worry about me eating down there. Think I'm too old."

"How old are you, anyway?"

"Oh, I don't know, about 82 or 84. Been in practice 63 years."

I began to have reservations about this Mexican lunch he was building up to. Had I known about his theories of driving a car, I would have been *more* concerned. But God never gives you more than you can take in one day.

"Real passion for good Mexican food, real passion. So what do you do when you've got a problem? First figure out where it comes from. Where's it come from in their case?"

"Eating onions and garlic."

"Eating it?"

"Yes, swallowing it."

"I used to think so, then I looked. Took garlic and onion, put it in large capsules and had people swallow them. No breath problem."

"I thought—"

"Then we inserted the capsules rectally—good absorption there you know—and again, no breath problem. Next I made a 'mash' of onion and garlic and painted it on the teeth. No odor. But! Just *touch* the tongue. There it is. Bad as can be. Well, once I figured out the problem the solution became clear. Clean the tongue. That wasn't as easy as I thought. Took several months and lots of trials. Only thing that worked was full-strength Clorox."

"Clorox!" I gasped.

"Full strength. Half strength didn't do a thing."

"Real Clorox, like for clothes?" I was still in shock.

"One and the same."

This one I didn't try until I got home. Full-strength Clorox—brother! Well, I tried it. Hot Mexican food complete with garlic guacamole and then the Clorox. I poured about a quarter of a teaspoon of it on my toothbrush, closed my eyes, stuck out my tongue—and—*what an experience.* Not bad—*certainly* not good. Unique. The first time it is a real surprise. After that, it's not so bad, and certainly worth it if you like Mexican food. No one will have to remind you to brush with regular toothpaste immediately after the Clorox job. Would you believe, after all this, he took me to a *Greek* restaurant?

That's where it really all started, in the Greek restaurant. It didn't take long for Harvey to get down to business. After briefly running through the time-honored causes of crooked teeth and improper facial development, he turned to his own studies in the twenties.

"As the twig is bent, so grows the tree."

"Yes?"

"Take that fellow over there—the waiter—he was slept on his back as a baby. Still does."

"Do you know the family well?"

"Nope." He had a clipped way of saying nope—almost as if it was only worth half a syllable. "Eat in here a lot, but I don't have to know him to tell how he sleeps. Know how lots of women sleep, and haven't slept with any of them."

I looked at the young—about 25—statuesque Greek—dark hair, dark eyes, two arms, two legs. What in the world had Harvey seen that I hadn't?

"Lookit."

I looked. "At what?"

"Fellow who just came in. Tummy sleeper. Written all over him."

Plaid suit, hat, brown shoes, six feet tall (so was the Greek), dark hair, dark eyes. I uncrossed my legs and crossed them the other way, picked up the menu, set it down, shuffled (patience is *not* my major virtue). I then put my elbow on the table, plopped my chin in my hand, and tried to speak slowly. "What on God's green earth are you *talking* about?"

"Bending twigs—bending people. When you sleep on your stomach you develop a stooped-over posture like that American fellow. Look at how his shoulder blades stick out like wings. Head's too far foward. When he turns toward us you'll see he has a narrow face."

"Know him?"

"Never saw him before."

"How come you know he has a narrow face?"

"Has to."

Where did I go wrong? I must have slept through a week of classes. "Look, I took three extra anatomy courses . . ."

"Lookit—he's turning."

Sure enough—he had a long, narrow face.

"So maybe his parents have long, narrow faces."

"You are thinking genetics. Read Price. He'll show you that changes in diet do the same thing to faces."

"Orthodontics—a dietary deficiency?"

My institutionalized training just collapsed. My brain started flashing little red lights that said, "Reject, reject—doesn't compute. Return to step one."

"My work. . ." Harvey was not aware of my turmoil, or chose to ignore it. He paused long enough for me to get on his train of thought. "My work has been to isolate the mechanical aspects of orthodontic causes. When you sleep on your face you are bending a twig."

"What do you mean, sleep on your face?" I pictured a face sticking nose first into a pillow.

"Tummy sleepers put pressure on their faces."

As if reading my mind he added, "Can't sleep nose down, so they turn so the total weight of their head is on one side of their face. This flattens the face on that side—or, if they turn now and again, it will flatten both sides of the face. That's how you get a long, narrow face."

"What does that do to the palate?"

"Ever take physics?"

"Yes."

"Then you tell me. Mother Nature's laws are pure, basic physics."

"Pushes it up and forms the *high narrow palatal vault.*" That I *had* heard in school. The high palate was associated with problems in the nasal cavities behind the nose. Crooked teeth went along with it too.

For the first time I began to see that his message was comprehensible; it was just that he had a 40-year head start on me.

"Say, he had a hand up there."

Here we go again. By now I was scribbling notes on my napkin.

"Put a hand under the face and you get more deformation. Cheek bones can't develop. Cross-bites can."

"Cross-bites?"

"You don't know what a cross-bite is?"

"Sure—that's where a lower tooth fits on the wrong side of an upper tooth when you close the teeth together."

Harvey frowned. "I'm not sure you could pass your dental exams with an explanation like that, but I know you know what it is. If a knuckle is under the face and it happens to habitually press on an upper tooth, the upper tooth moves inward."

"I get the idea. I was just thinking of a quite *simple* two-tooth cross-bite I tried to correct in school. Two molars were in cross-bite. I banded each, hooked a rubber band between them and sat back. Sure enough—in three months they were in proper relationship to each other, so I removed the bands. Six months later—zing. A cross-bite case for next year's seniors. It relapsed."

"Took off one orthodontic appliance and left the other."

"What other?"

"The hand. The hand, head, fingers, knuckles, arm, pillow, all these things are orthodontic appliances. Only they work *against* you. That's why the Greek boy has such a beautiful physique. Look at his posture. Most people call it regal, or proud. I call it a typical back sleeper's posture. You know, kids only grow when they are asleep."

"No, I didn't know that."

"That's why they sleep a lot. That's why it's so important to sleep them in the position you want them to develop in. Back sleepers develop bilaterally. Most muscles have counterparts—right and left. How can an athelete develop properly if one side develops less than the other? Only when a kid is on his back can things develop with equal vigor. Tummy sleepers mess up their spine, so does the side sleeper. Only the back sleeper has a straight back. Faces are the same way. Only on the back can your genetic laws have full effect. Mash those faces and you have crooked teeth, crooked noses, undeveloped cheek bones, small lower jaws, receding chins—even visual problems."

"Visual?"

My mind raced to analyze all previous comments and beat him to the punch. Ding, like a typewriter turned loose by the tabulator and nothing's set. Scan-bam! Nothing. My mind didn't find one thing to register.

"Opthalmologists agree with me," Harvey was saying, "say it makes sense. Never did anything with it though. If you put pressure on the side of the face—say with a hand under a pillow—there is pressure on the side of the skull. This prevents the orbit from developing to its full roundedness. Result? An eye that's not fully rounded. They call it astigmatism.

"Primitive people knew the art of child rearing. That's why they swaddled their kids. That's why the Indians had cradleboards. Primitives were more concerned about their kids than we are. Made a big thing about it. When young people wanted to marry they were put on special diets so their babies would be healthy. In some tribes you were not allowed to have sex with your wife until your baby was two years old. Why? So that mother could recuperate and have another healthy baby. Healthy babies were the key to survival of the tribe.

"That's where you come in, Huggins. You ought to study the primitives. Learn ancient wisdom. Won't hurt you. I've heard you speak before groups. You're okay. Come across in a way that people like to listen. Do something with that talent. Give people something worth listening to. Find out how we can adopt primitive customs and adapt them to modern living. We can't go back—but you can go forward."

My mind was excited. I knew I had to do what he said. I didn't need to know *why* anymore, I just knew it had to be done.

Chapter Three

Why Raise Bent Bodies?

Just how do sleeping habits affect normal growth? Pictorially, you can follow the destruction of beauty by improper pressures.

An old physician once told me, "you will never be able to recognize the abnormal 'til you know what's normal." That's a good philosophy for beauty. When we learn to recognize what constitutes beauty, then we will know what causes ugliness.

Posture is one of the first things we notice about people. It's what gives people "character." Look at the silhouette of the boy on the left in figure 3. He looks pretty good. Note the flat tummy and form of the back. Note the slight curve from his shoulder to his waist to his hips. His head is centered over his body. Do people actually look like that? Look at Eric on the right, in figure 4. He just stepped up, turned to the side and we took his picture. No effort was made to pose him. Mother Nature strikes a pose of beauty when allowed to grow and develop properly.

Look at Eric face on and from the back in figures 5 and 6. He stands straight. There is no tilt to his head one way or the other, and his shoulders are at the same level. Notice how symmetrical he is. This is beauty.

Now let's look at the posture of the tummy sleeper, on the right in figure 7. Notice how prominent his shoulder blades are. Look at the increased curve from his shoulder blade to his hip. His head is tipped slightly forward, and it is not centered over his body. His stomach sticks out a bit even though he is thin. Compare the back and tummy sleepers. Which posture would you prefer for your son?

Figure 8 is an old photograph of an outstanding set of "wings." This girl's shoulder blades strike an outstanding pose. Some people have commented that her head is facing the wrong way.

Heads are the next thing we notice. Remember that the first part of the head to calcify is the occiput, the little knob you can feel on the back of your head. If the weight of the head does *not* rest here during sleep, this area experiences an *overgrowth,* while the thin, slightly calcified "membrane bones" of the face collapse under the head's weight. The resultant underdeveloped chin signifies a small lower jaw that will *not* be able to properly house all the lower teeth, as shown by the silhouette on the right in figure 9.

Do you think this can't happen? Check on some two- and three-year-olds you know, and look at them from the side (figure 10).

Looking down on a person from above, you can easily see developmental differences between a back sleeper and a tummy sleeper. Here again, in figure 11, you can see the forward set of the head and the jutting shoulder blades of the tummy sleeper versus the stately appearance of the back sleeper. The back sleeper certainly presents a more pleasing appearance than the tummy sleeper, doesn't he?

I nearly hung from the ceiling by my heels to get this photo (figure 12), but it was worth the effort. Note where the center of his body should be—through the shoulders—and you can get an idea of how far out of symmetry he is.

Side sleepers are fairly easy to identify because of the distinct "finger prints" they create on themselves. Look at this fellow's back (figure 13). The drawing visualizes how the spine is encouraged to develop with one long curve in it.

Look again and note the position of the lower shoulder blade. It protrudes. If you run your hand across the back of a side sleeper, you will feel one shoulder blade sticking out. This is a dead give away of side sleeping, but not the only evidence.

Look at the face-on view of the side sleeper in figure 14. A side sleeper's hands have to get into the act. Sometimes one, sometimes *both* are under the pillow putting that much more pressure against the developing face. After adulthood hands around the face can still move teeth. They do it much more slowly, but it can still cause a problem. If a dentist has just placed a new bridge and the patient sleeps with a hand touching that area, the pressure can move the teeth slightly. This is noted by the

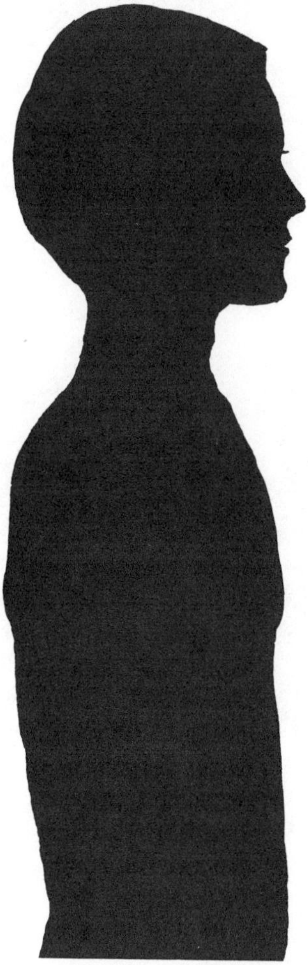

Figure 3

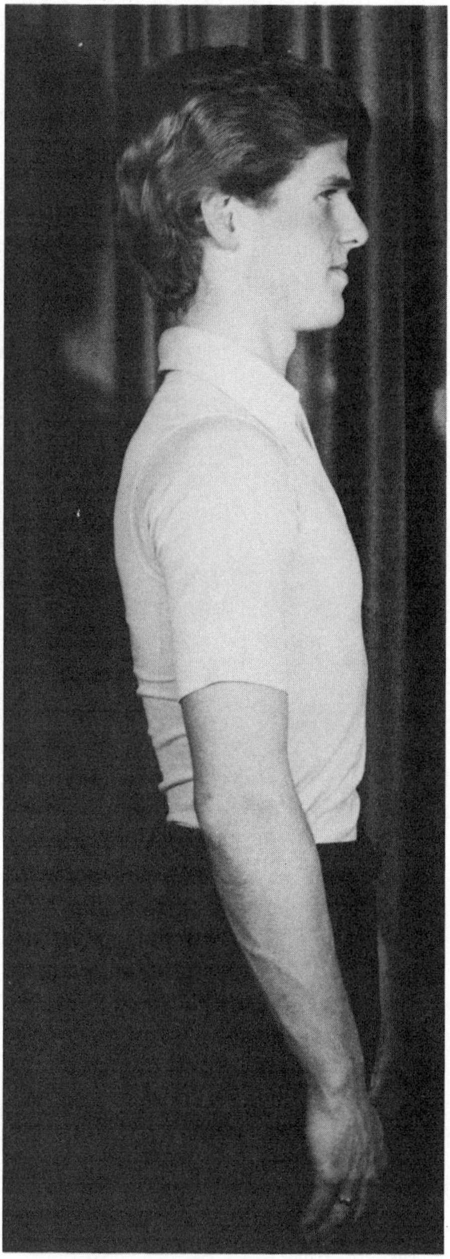

Figure 4

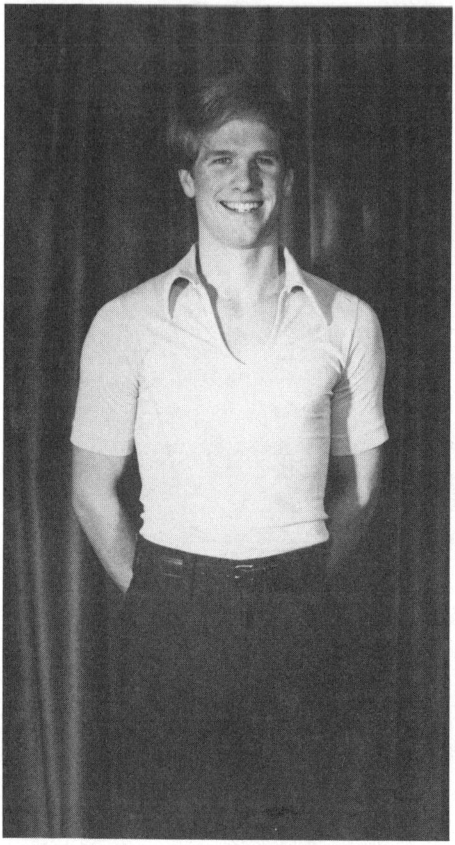

Figure 5

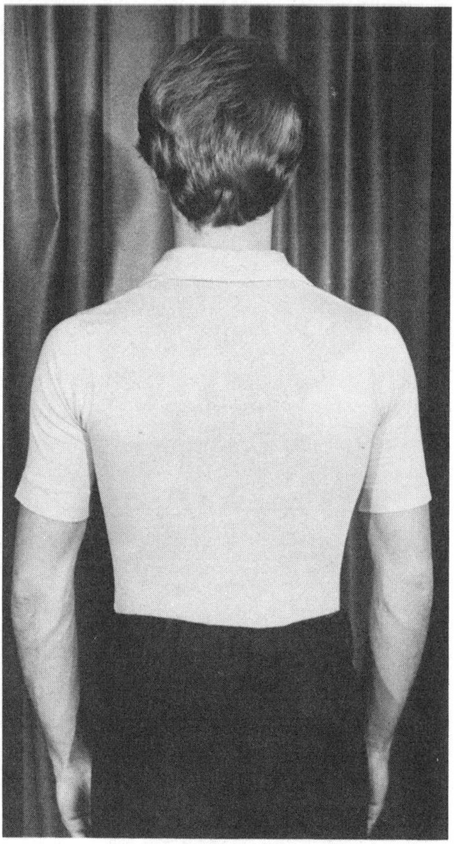

Figure 6

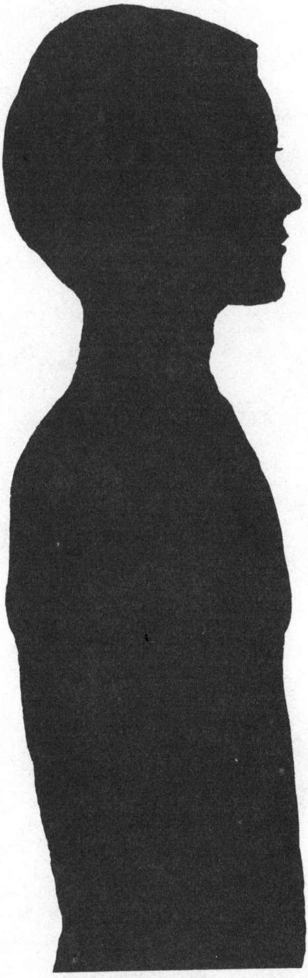

Figure 3

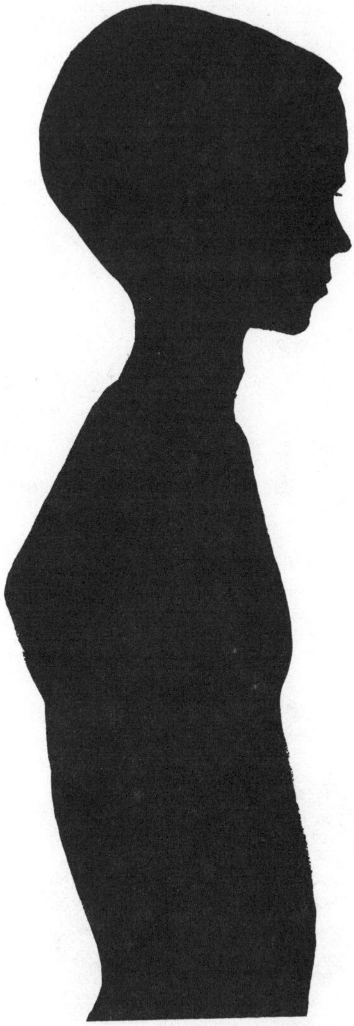

Figure 7

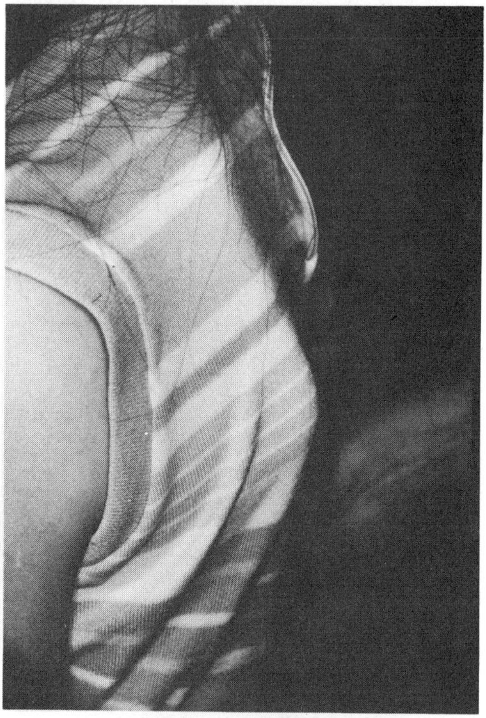

Figure 8

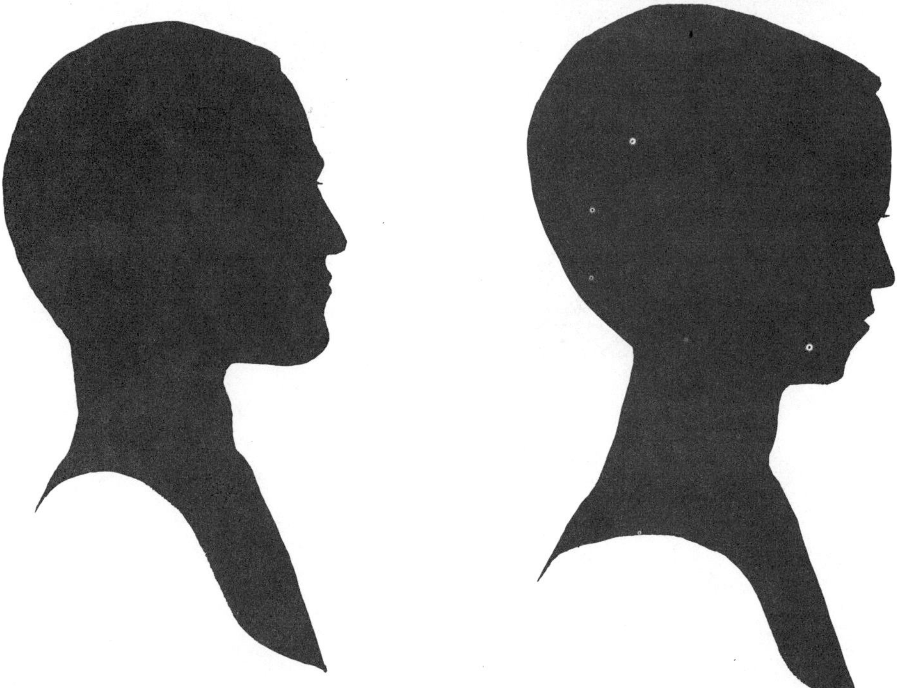

Figure 9

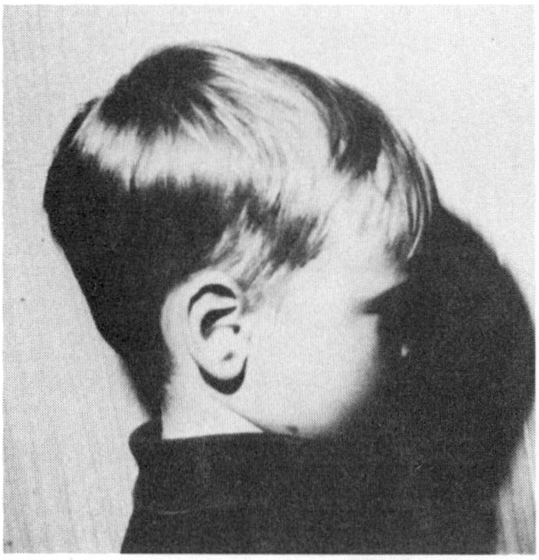

Figure 10

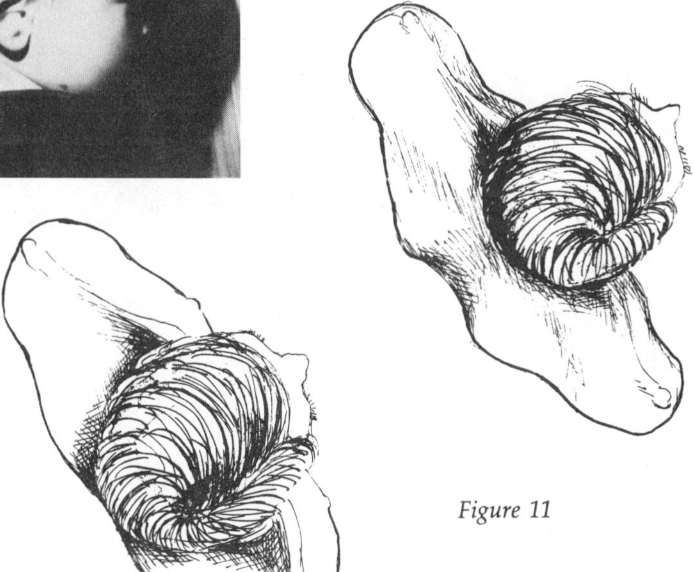

Figure 11

Figure 12

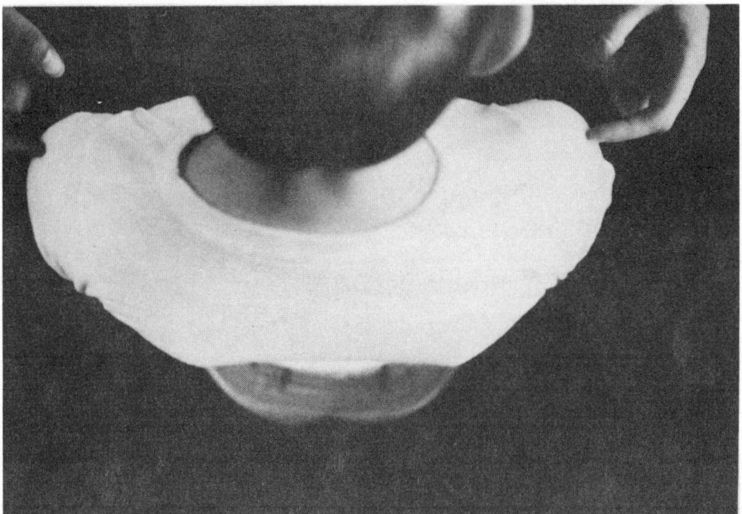

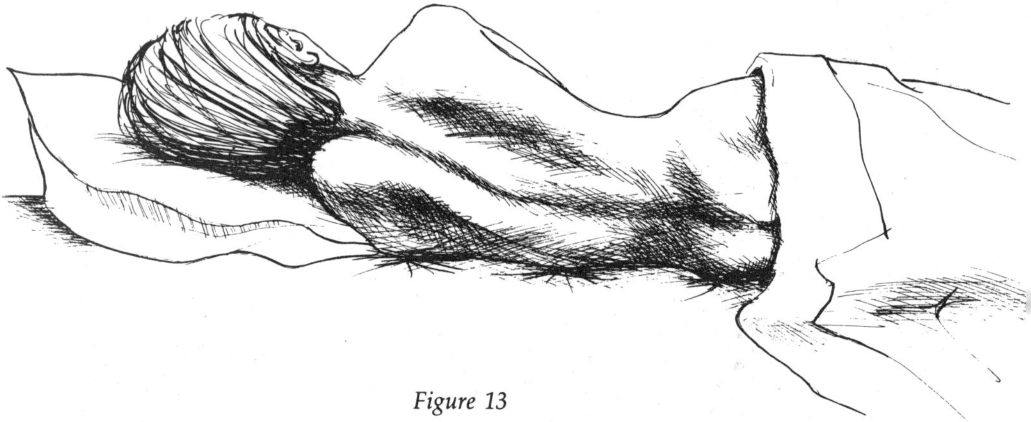

Figure 13

Figure 14

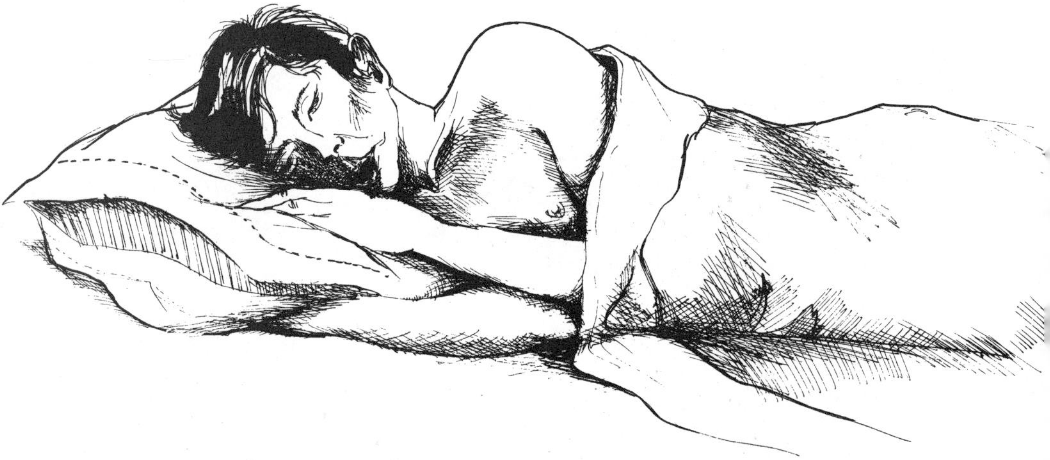

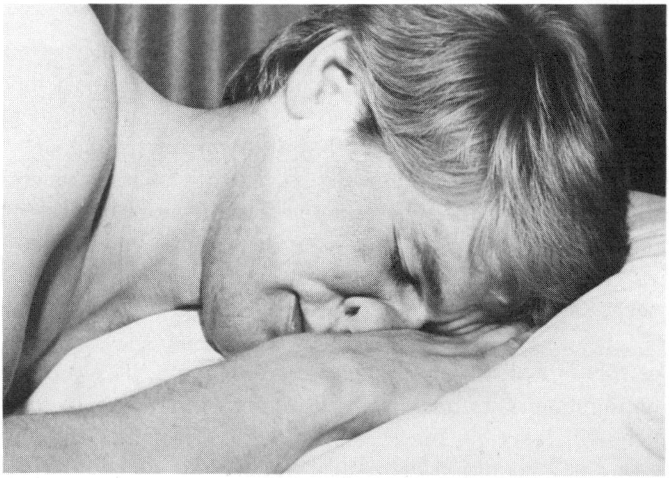

Figure 15

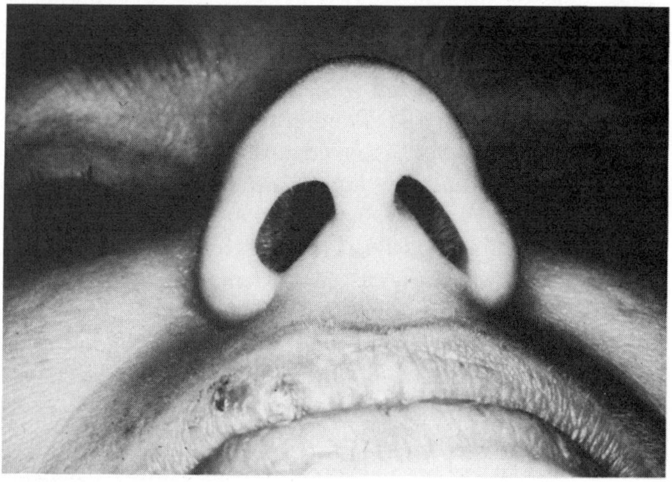

Figure 16

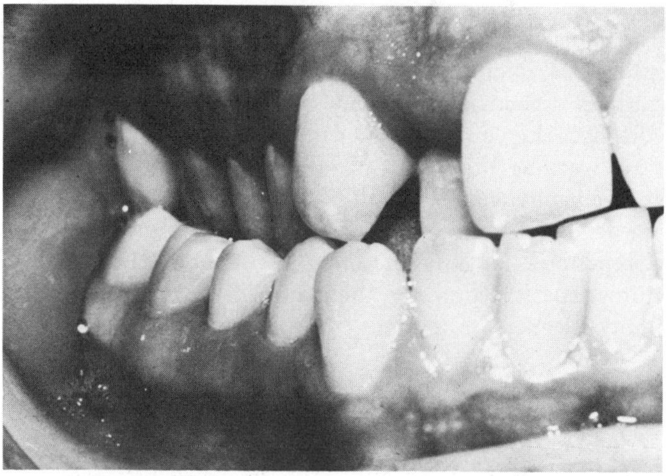

Figure 17

patient because it creates a "high spot" on the bridge. The dentist adjusts it, the patient sleeps on it a few more nights, and bingo—we have another high spot. These movements may be only a hundredth of an inch, but the result is very irritating to both the patient and the doctor.

If the side sleeper turns his face a few degrees so that his hand touches his nose (figure 15), his nose changes shape. You may not often be in a position to look at people's noses, but as a dentist I have had many "opportunities" to look at lots of them. In figure 16, is what you may never have seen. Grotesque! It couldn't happen. Oh? Gaze on this schnoz.

A nose like this is a dead giveaway of crooked teeth. The problem teeth will be in the molars, or back teeth. Pressure enough to distort the nose this much will leave its mark on the teeth. The most common distortion we find is a condition called *cross-bite.* This is the term applied when the upper teeth are tucked inside the lowers. The uppers should overlap the lowers. In figure 17 you can see a normal condition in the smaller teeth (bicuspids) and a cross-bite in the molars.

Incidently, the whole nose gets moved in this sleeping position—not just the nostrils. Photographs don't show crooked noses well, but, take my word for it, crooked noses are ugly.

Since both the human head and clay are somewhat plastic, I had an artist, Wade Webster, make two clay heads for me. Starting with a perfectly good head (figure 18), he applied a little orthodontic force to the nose (figures 19 and 20) and ended up with a nasal septum deviation —or crooked nose (figure 21).

Make a fist and we have a real orthodontic device (figure 22). This creates a weird-looking mouth because the bicuspid area (midway back) is narrow, while the front teeth and molars at the back are quite wide (figure 23).

The real problem creator is the tummy sleeper. Tummy sleeping starts out to be so cute. Many mommies and grandmommies have smiled and giggled when the object of their affections kicks its little hind end up in the air. "Isn't he cute?" No, it is an act of survival, not theatrics. Babies are "belly breathers." You can see a sway beginning in the back (figure 24). This predisposes the young charmer to middle-age back problems. Three curves are working their way into this child's developing spine. None will help him in any way.

Now the fun begins. Tummy sleepers are the most *creative* sleepers. Their massive repertoire has only one thing in common. The orthodontist. Actually, if we speak technically, there are two problems developing in young tummy sleepers, orthodontic *and* orthopedic. Orthodontic problems are those limited to tooth positions. Orthopedic problems are those limited to bone. Unfortunately, the bones we are watching contain teeth—therefore, we have an overlapping orthodontic-orthopedic problem. The tummy sleeper excels all other sleepers in his ability to distort facial bones and interfere with growth patterns. He does this by laying antibeauty factors around his face. They include hands, arms and pillows. Let's look at some favorite tummy sleeping positions and the problems they foster.

We'll start with the *stacker.* He folds his pillow and arms together into a four-story force system—two arms and two layers of pillow, as in figure 25.

This may not do much harm to the face, but it puts so much pressure against the head that it is forced out of its mid-line position. These sleepers are easily identified by the tilt of their heads when they face you. (See figure 26.)

Bringing the hand into action as shown in figure 27 prevents total development of that cheekbone. This is shown also in the clay figure from a top-of-the-head view, figure 28. Note that the right cheekbone is more prominent than the left. This means less bone development and loss of facial symmetry. Ugly. This problem is fairly high up on the face and may not mess up the teeth. Just the face.

Now let's move the hand down an inch. As shown in figure 29, the knuckles are in good position to create the "blocked-out cuspid" (figure 30). The cuspid is also known as the "eye tooth." Pressure here reduces the growth potential on *one side* of the dental arch and *not* on the other. Sleepers have a habitual favorite position and spend the majority of their sleeping time there. This was suggested by Harvey and by monitoring the "sleeping machine that stays awake all night." This machine has a position sensor that records one of eight basic head positions while a person sleeps. The position shown in figure 29 frequently creates the condition illustrated in figure 30.

Let's drop that hand down about an inch and a half and see what happens (figure 31). Here pressure is against the *lower* teeth. Pressure here can stunt some of the growth of the lower jaw, leading to a smaller chin. That's an orthopedic problem. It can also move a lower tooth inward toward the tongue so that it doesn't function properly with the upper teeth. That's an orthodontic problem (figure 32).

Mashing the nose is not limited to the side sleeper. The old wrestling hold—the full Nelson—can influence your nose. Not only that, but look at the neck-to-body relationship in figure 33. Any wonder why some tummy sleepers wake up with a stiff neck?

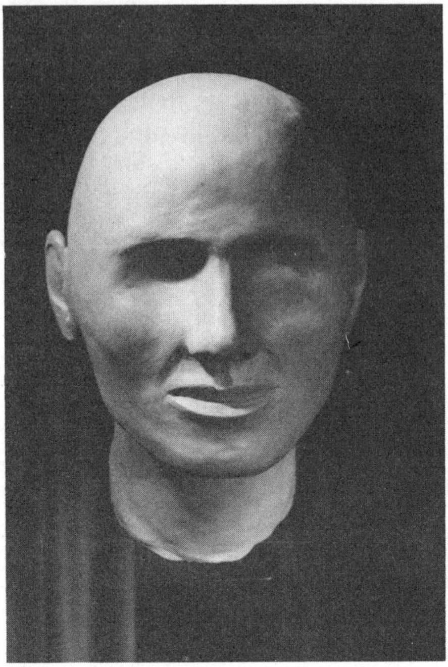
Figure 18

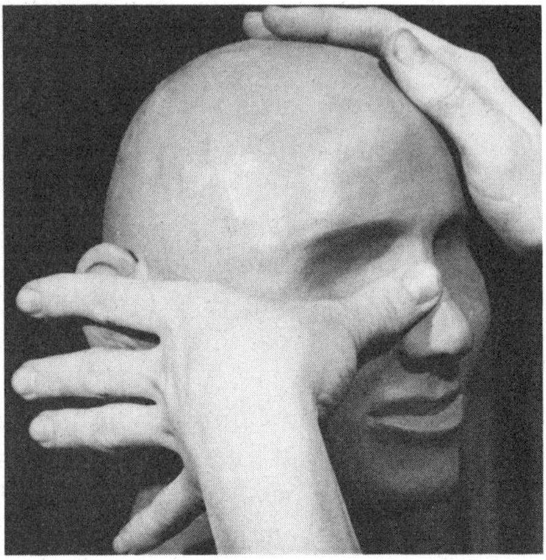
Figure 19

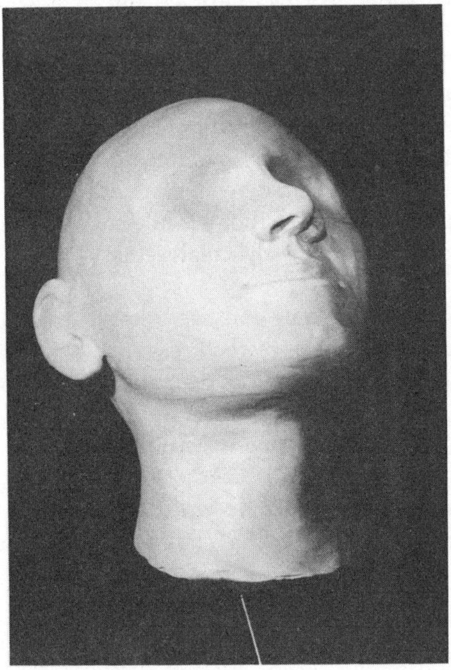
Figure 20

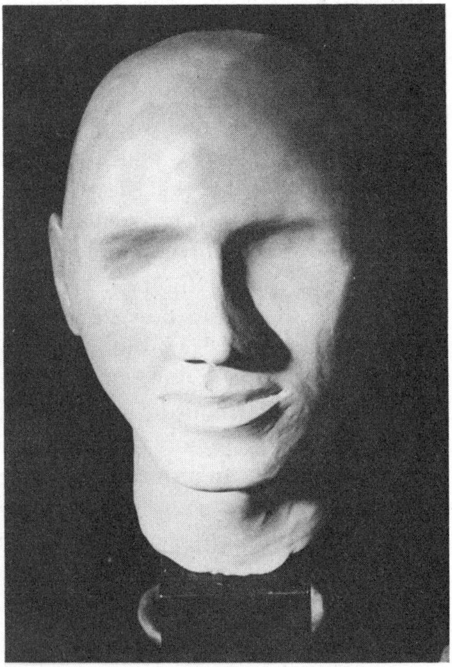
Figure 21

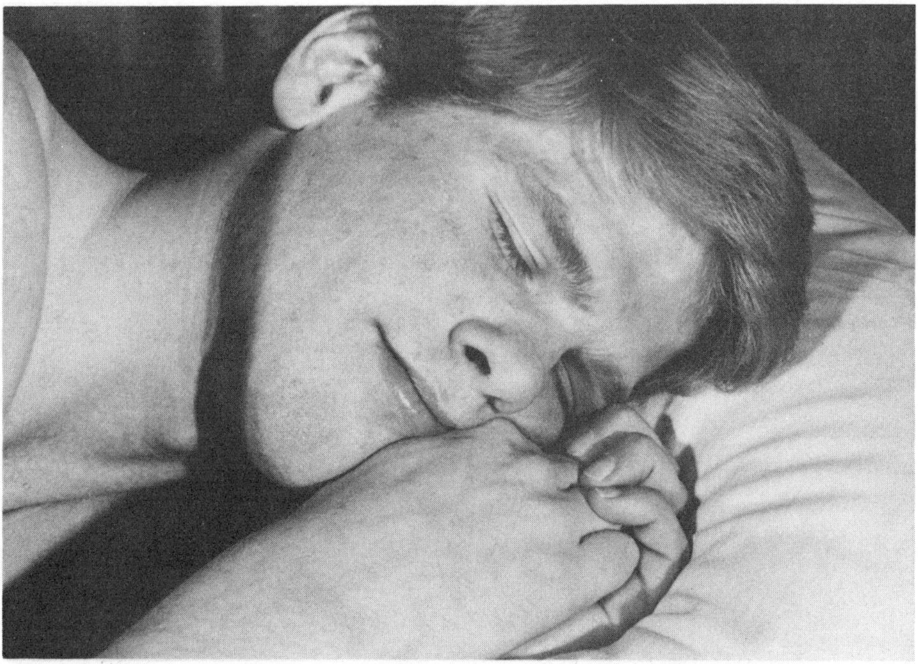

Figure 22

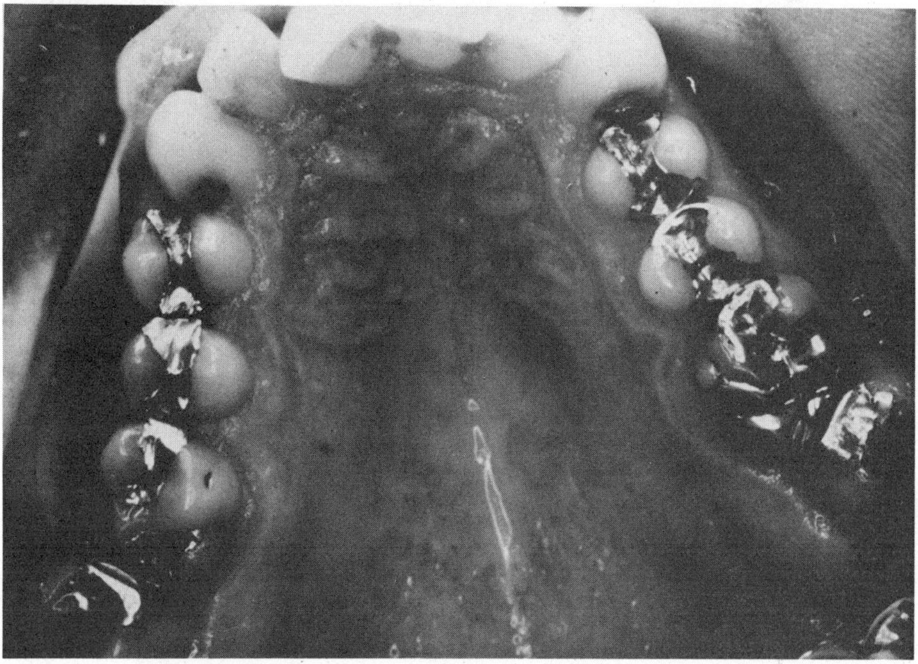

Figure 23

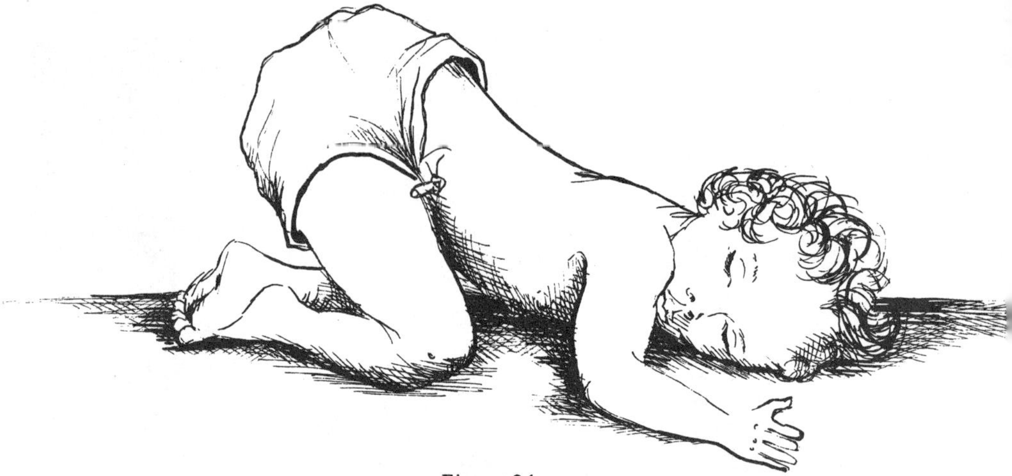

Figure 24

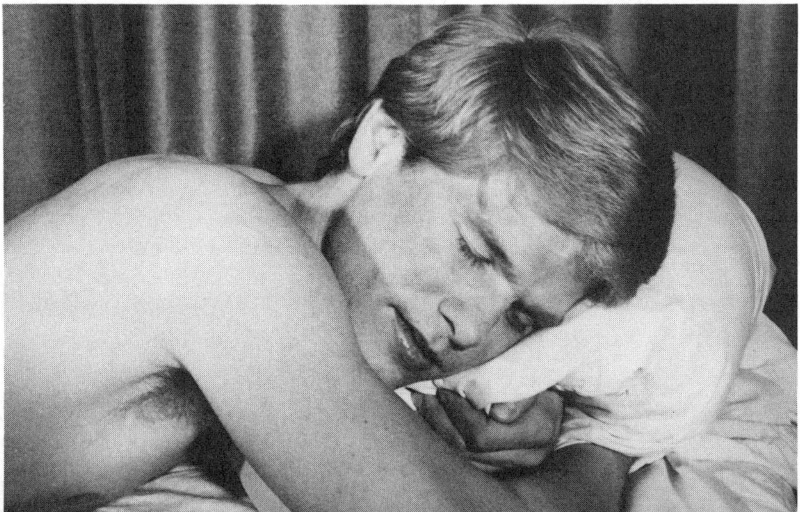

Figure 25

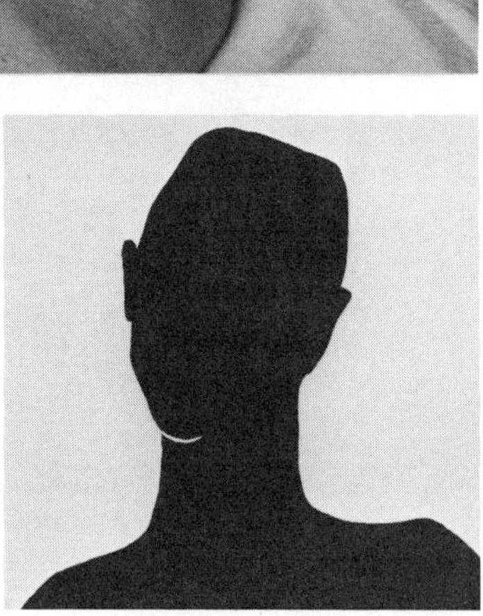

Figure 26

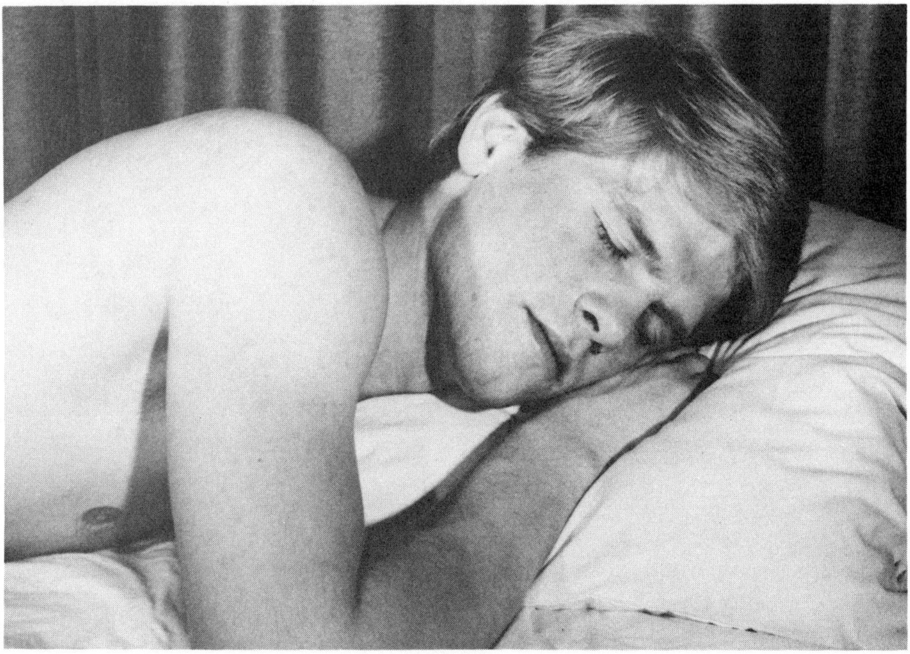

Figure 27

Figure 28

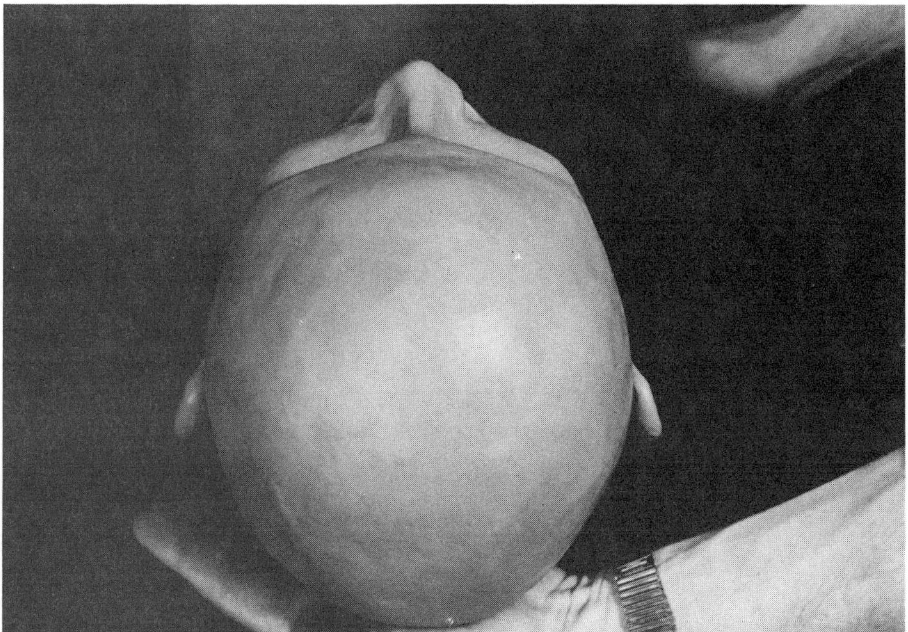

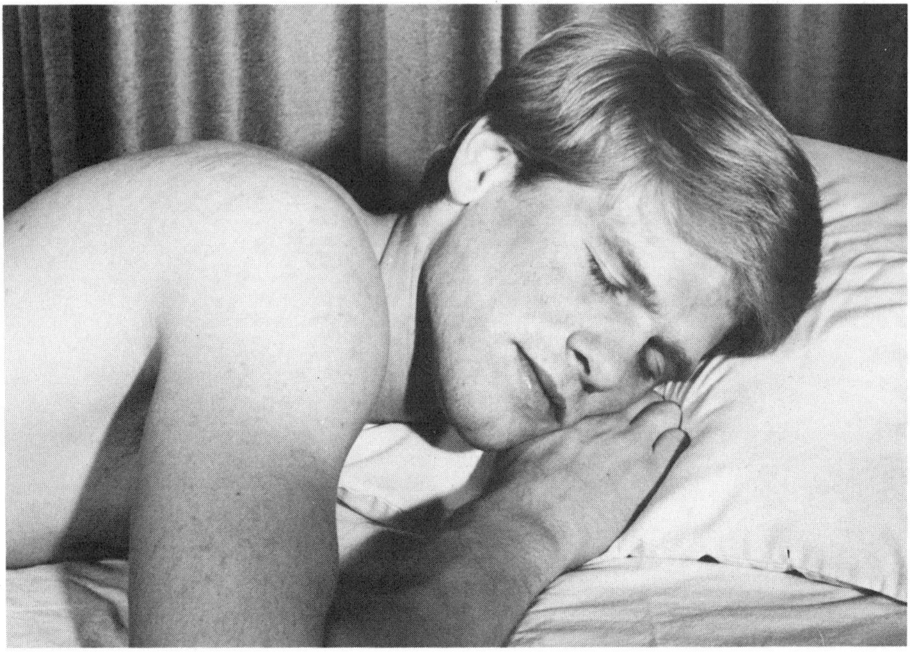

Figure 29

Figure 30

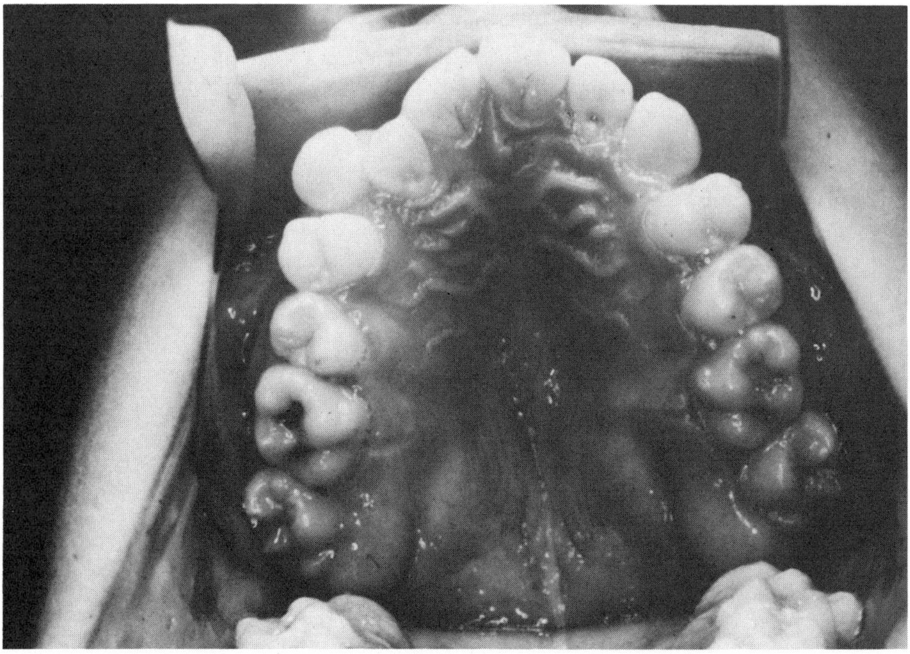

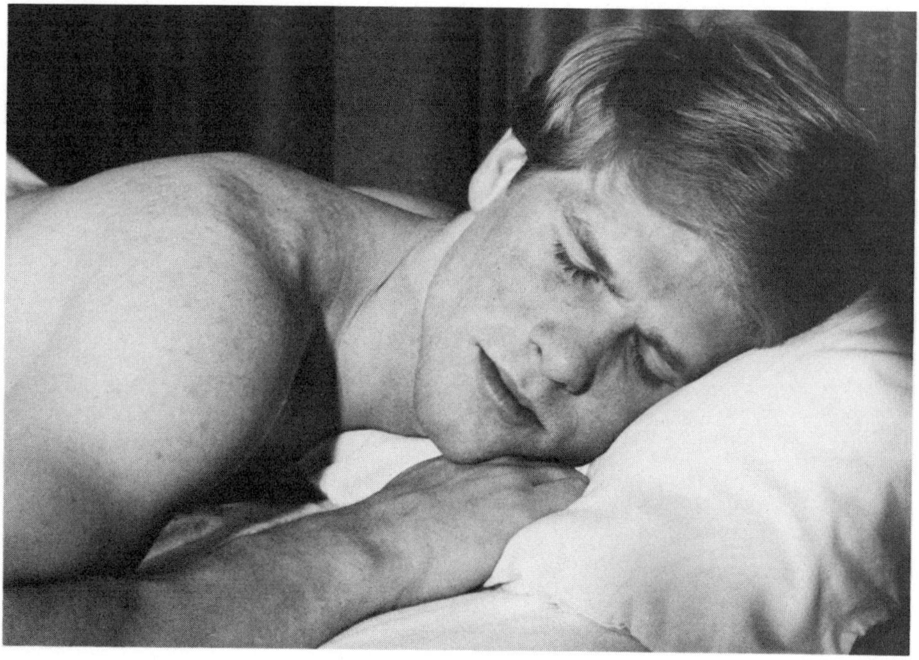

Figure 31

Figure 32

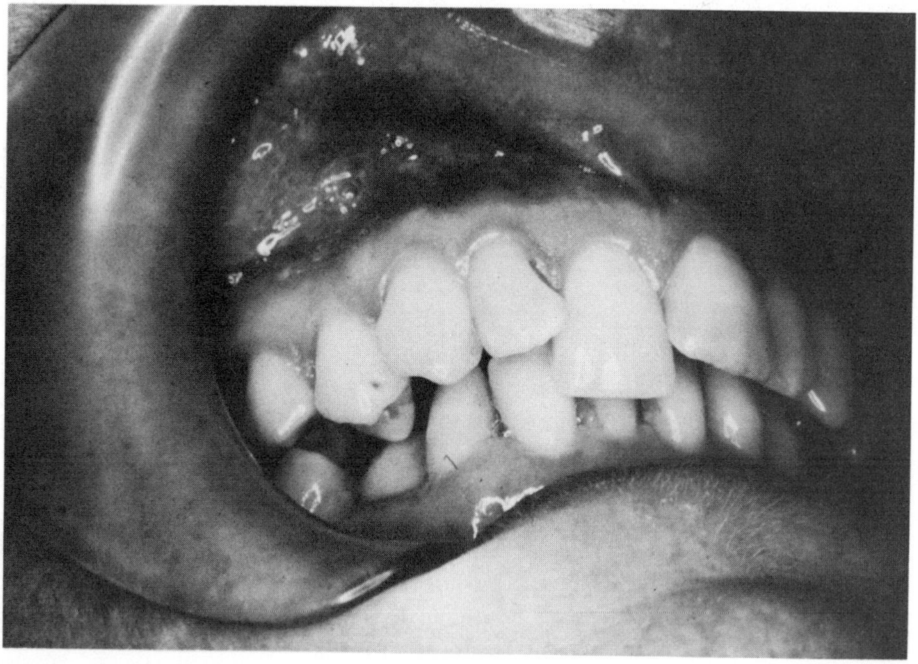

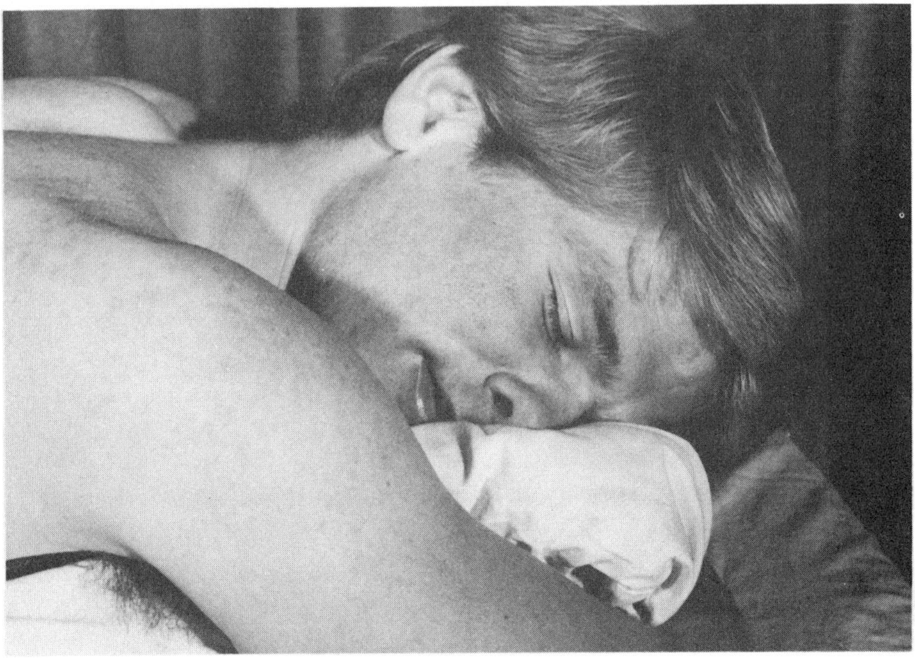

Figure 33

Figure 34

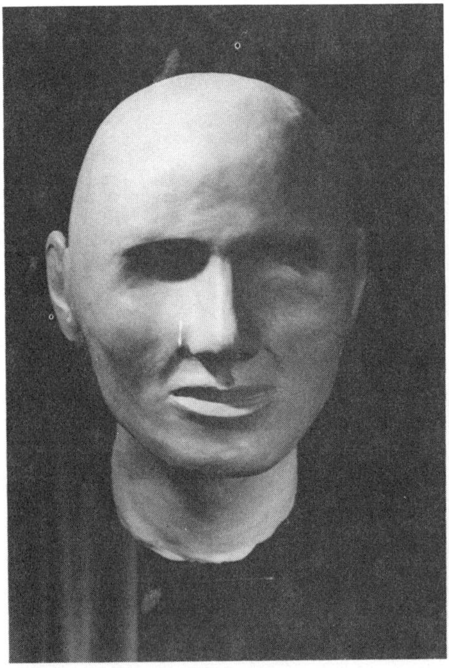

Figure 35

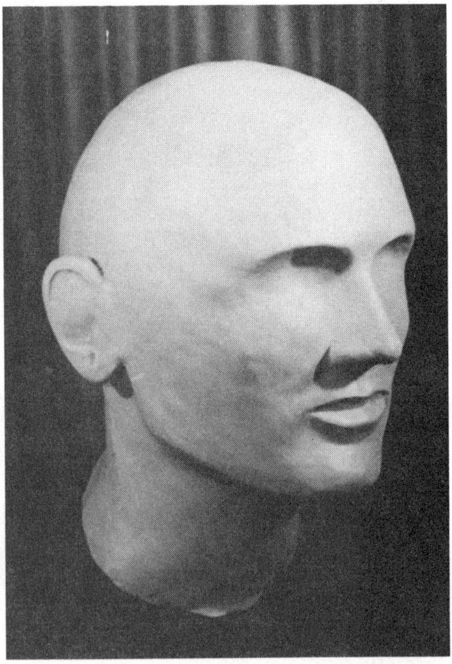

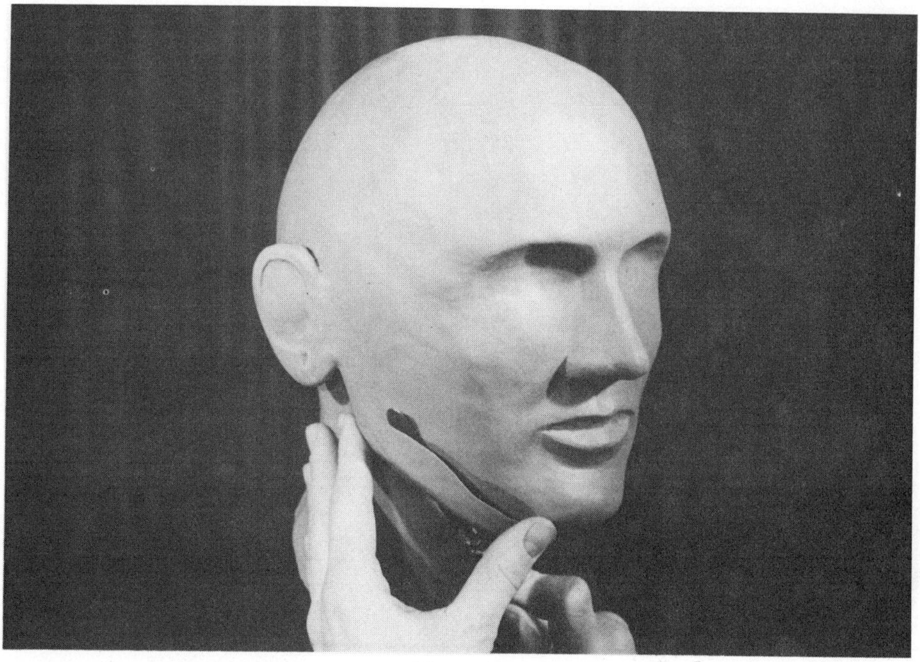

Figure 36

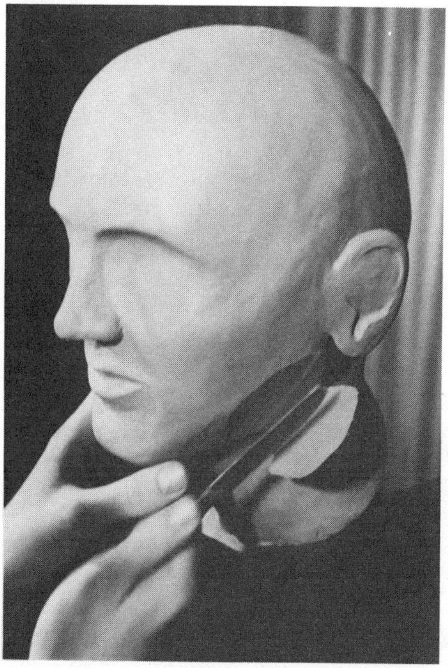

Figure 37

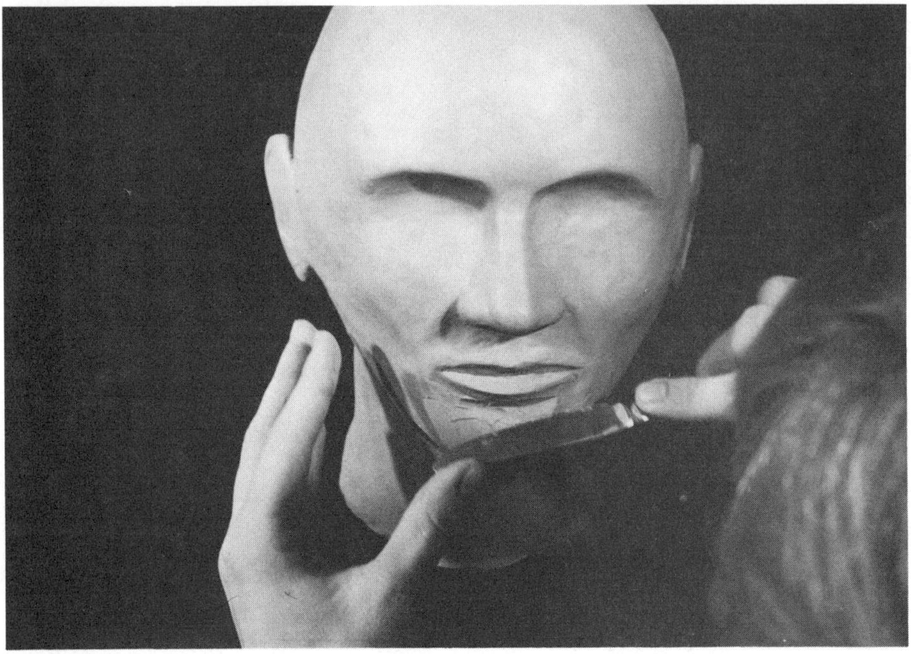

Figure 38

Figure 39

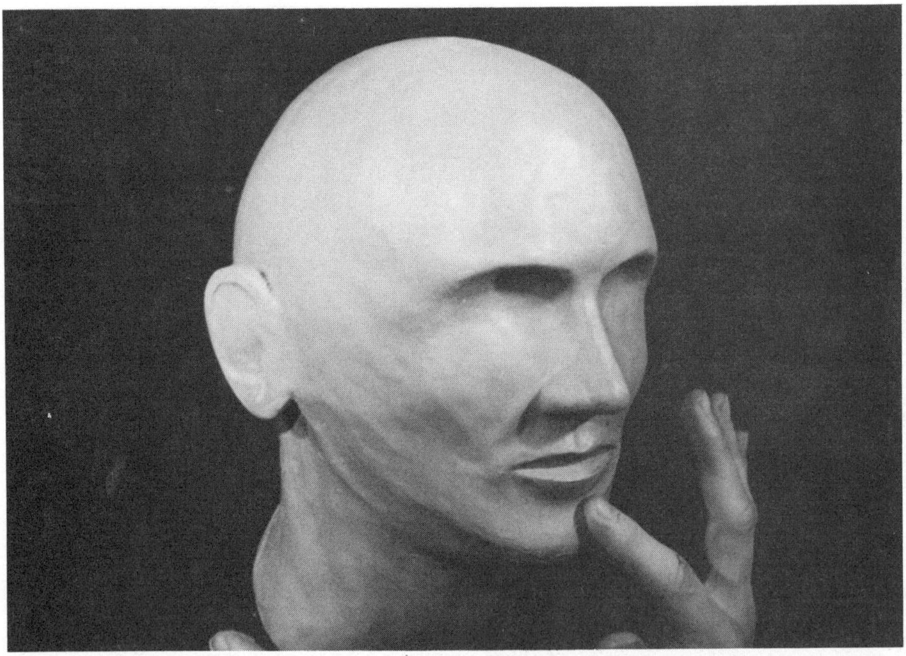

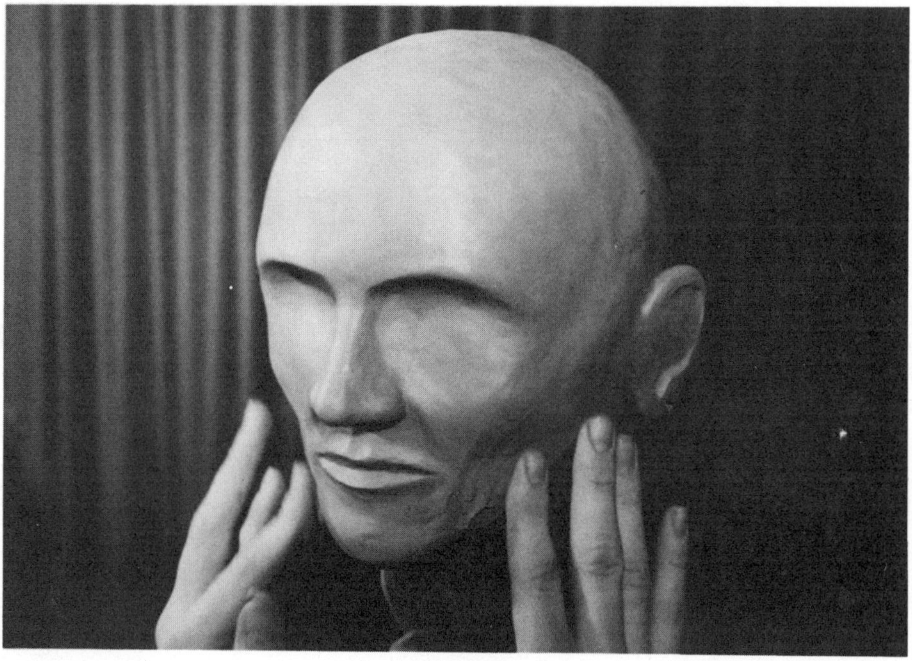

Figure 40

Figure 41

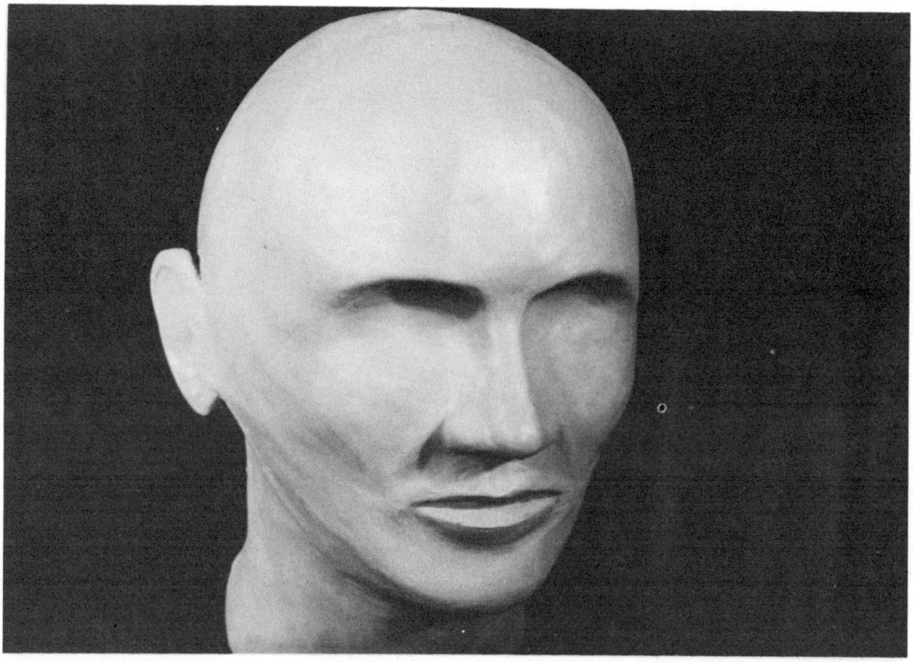

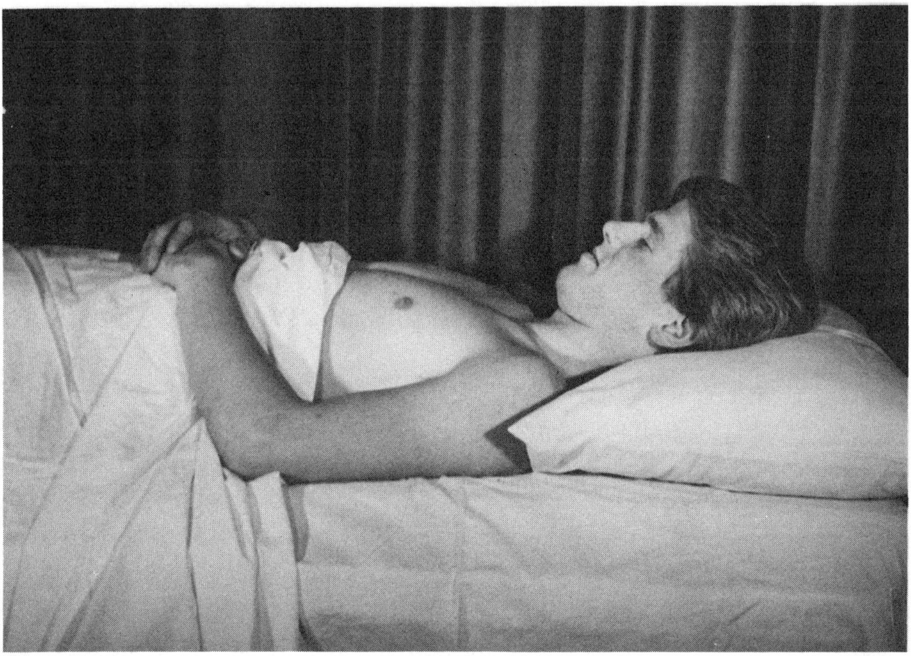

Figure 42

Figure 43

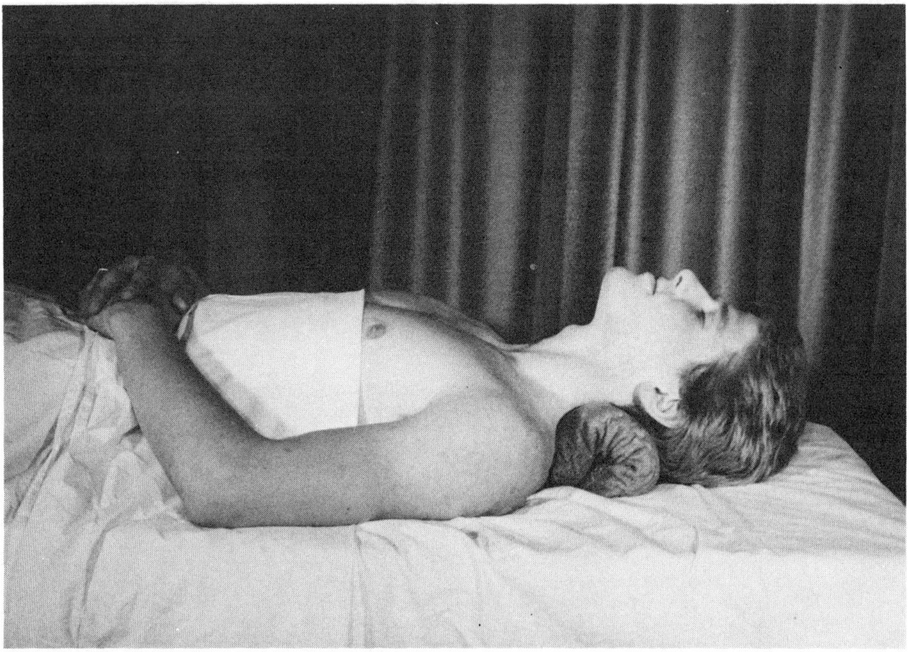

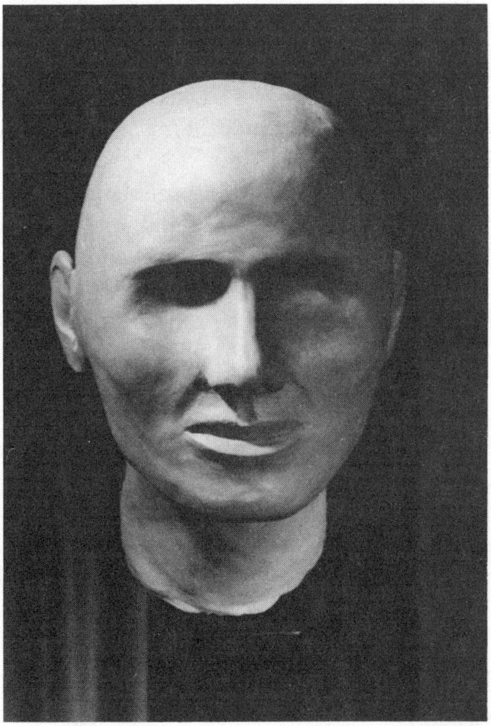
Figure 44

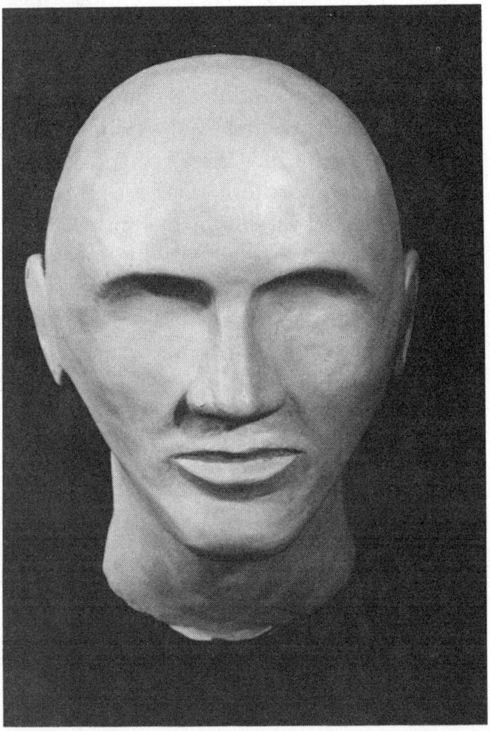
Figure 45

Let's grow a bit older—say into the third or fourth decade. What's the biggest fear to both men and women? Wrinkles! Look closely above Eric's left eye in figure 33. What's being formed here? The position shown is also good for forming wrinkles on the chin.

How about a time-lapse look at the tummy sleeping problem with the clay head as our model? What changes are we really making? We can start with a perfectly good head as in the model in figures 34 and 35.

Tummy sleeping will narrow the face. Mechanically, this position prevents the genetic potential from fulfilling its role. In figure 36 the artist is removing some of the genetic potential, stunting it by the application of pressure.

Next, we can see in figure 37 what happens when a hand is under the face. The area removed here is growth potential that would have supplied plenty of room for the wisdom teeth to come in.

Tummy sleepers also fall short of developing a full chin. To illustrate, Wade removes some of the chin in figure 38. In figures 39 and 40 he refines the chin and blends the changes brought about by sleeping habits into a final form (figure 41).

How should you sleep? From all of these observations, sleeping on your back wins out as the overall best position (figure 42). Pressures are evenly distributed on bones that can stand stress; paired sets of muscles are the same length (remember, you grow when you are asleep); and because back sleepers move less during the night, you probably rest better in that position.

But what about snoring? Yes, in figure 42 everything is fine—except for producing the tendency to snore. Why? The pillow. Look how Eric's head is tipped by the pillow. This neck position *can* make one snore. Not always, but the predisposition is *definitely* there. A simple solution (good for both your sleeping partner and the neck) is to use a small pillow, as shown in figure 43. The pillow needs to be large enough to support the spine in your neck but *that's all.* Your head should be in line with the rest of your body.

Most ancient cultures—Chinese, Japanese, African, Indian—had small "cervical" pillows. Cervical is the name applied to that portion of the spine in the neck. They had super bodies and great postures. It is interesting to note that the orientals used small *wooden* pillows. Eric is *not* on a wooden pillow. He is using a pillow made from a washcloth folded, sewn together and filled with polyurethane foam. A tube sock stuffed firmly with foam and seamed at the end works well for many people. It is quick and easy to make.

Dr. Karl Nishimura, a California orthodontist, recently told me his relatives sent him a wooden pillow from Japan. In his culture, if a relative sends you a gift, you use it. He was pretty uncomfortable the first few nights because of one spot in particular. It rubbed. He thought about whittling the pillow down, but didn't. Within a few more nights he was comfortable and had fewer neck problems. He wasn't really aware of the slight neck pain he had had for years until this wooden pillow straightened out his cervical spine and the pain went away.

All genetics aside, many familial facial characteristics are the result of similar sleeping habits. Look at the before and after pictures in figure 44 and 45. You've seen them both. They both look like people we see every day on any street. Remember, genetics—our inheritance—is only as strong as we let it be. It is potential, what *can* happen. If we don't feed genetics properly, it falls short of the mark. If we put mechanical pressure on our faces, our genetics can't push back hard enough, and through no fault of our own we become Ugly Kids.

Chapter Four

How Our Ancestors Formed Full Faces

Most peoples of the world before 1800 grew beautiful kids. Though their reasons differed, they all used essentially the same methods. Their techniques horrify the modern American mother.

I was planning to attend a meeting in Arizona within six weeks, so I decided it would be a good idea to drive and make some stops at museums on the way. Things fell into place during the next two weeks while I sought out "child cultures" in the local libraries. This search led me to the anthropology department at Colorado College in Colorado Springs, where the staff gave me the names of anthropologists who were working in museums in New Mexico and Arizona. Two of my friends in Albuquerque, Den and Barb Micheel, rummaged through some local library books on the Indian cultures, and soon I became barraged with unassociated material. I stored away many isolated tidbits—some useful within days—others within years. Others are still sitting in my mind just being interesting isolated tidbits.

Den and Barb found many studies about Indians and whites living in the same area. Then Den came up with a piece of information that amazed me. He found notes from the Louis and Clark expedition that continually made reference to the beautiful stature of the Indians. Each new tribe merited a postural comment, but it was consistent. Indians were pretty people. I figured they had to be *outstanding* for these men who were trained to chart rivers and mountain ranges to remark so frequently about a subject not related to topography.

I recalled what Harvey Stallard had said about beautiful postures. It seemed that posture and crooked teeth had a connection, and that the foundation for both was laid down before people are two years old. Where were these Indians the first two years of life? On cradleboards. For the majority of the first year of life they were strapped to cradleboards nearly 23 hours a day. This could be good—could be bad. I decided to study cradleboards.

One fine Sunday morning I drove up to a New Mexico museum and started looking in windows. There it was! The most beautiful cradleboard I had ever seen. Big. It must have belonged to someone of rank in the tribe. It had a large beaded mat that extended several feet out all the way around. It might have been a ceremonial rug; I had never seen such a thing written up. There were reflections in the window which made photography nearly impossible. I focused as well as I could through the window, and as the cradleboard came into focus, I could see an Indian face in it. I looked up from the camera and found that the face had a body and legs and a broom, which it was waving in a disconcerting fashion. We faced off at the glass door and stared at each other. I had a flashback to Stallard. Perhaps I should have taken that six weeks to learn a language.

"I want a picture."

"I know. Come back Monday."

"I'll be gone Monday. Can't you just unlock the door for a minute? I'll take the picture and leave?"

"Call man," he said, tapping on a card taped to the corner of the window. I recognized the name as one given to me by a Colorado College professor.

* * *

"Did you attend Colorado College in Colorado Springs?"

"Why, yes, but how did you know?"

I identified my contact, and the museum director couldn't wait to come down and show his establishment. The whole thing, 5,000 square feet! I spent an hour behind iron bars in the vault looking at old pawn turquoise jewelry. I saw pots from the year one and lots of Indian artifacts.

"Hey, you ought to see Dr. Christy Turner at Tempe," my host announced as we came out of the vault. "He was telling me a few weeks ago that he was advisor to someone studying cradleboards."

As I headed for Tempe, Arizona, it dawned on me that in all the excitement I had forgotten to find out about the fancy cradleboard.

* * *

"Hate people who try to take advantage of deformed folks," Christy Turner said, looking over his glasses at me. I felt he was trying to look older than I by wearing a moustache and scowling. He chewed his pipe and scowled again. I buttoned my coat and put my hands behind my back. This always made me look older. Neither of us had reached 35.

"Always suspicious of graduate students trying to hurt someone."

"I'm not a graduate student."

"Who's paying for your research?"

"No one."

"Where did you get the money for your trip?"

"Me."

"Why?"

" 'Why' what?"

"Why are you studying without getting paid?"

"I'm interested."

"You ought to get a government grant."

"I can't. I'm not working for a university."

"That's stupid. Ought to let the government do it."

He finally took my name and local motel address. A few hours later I got a call from a Margaret Bodine. She had done things right. She had a government grant.

"Doctor, I simply must talk with you. Dr. Turner tells me you are an authority on Indian cradleboards."

Alas! Six weeks of my study and I'm an authority. Boy, did I fool Turner. It turned out that Margaret knew a lot more about cradleboards than I did, but she talked faster and I never had the opportunity to divulge my ignorance. She provided me with much needed information, but it didn't find its slot until several weeks later. Margaret was concerned about the high incidence of hip dysplasia (a congenital deformity of the hip that makes one walk with a limp) among the White Mountain Apaches. She was going to use a pressure gauge in cradleboards to see if the swaddling practices could be implicated in the development of this malady. She and a group of orthopedic surgeons were going to study three generations of these Apaches. The orthopedic doctors felt that heredity could be responsible.

Ronnie Lupe, the White Mountain Apache tribal chairman, had told Margaret that some 60 percent of the children were kept on cradleboards for seven to nine months. This is what turned her on. She felt that the cradleboard could be responsible for the hip problems. By this time I was feeling possessive about cradleboards and hoped that they weren't the offenders. How could something that was good for so many Indians on the Louis and Clark trail be so damaging to the Apaches? I had only to keep my eyes open and listen a little longer.

While driving through The Square in Santa Fe, New Mexico, I spotted the most beautiful specimen of mankind I had ever seen. Fully six foot two, 200 pounds and a posture that stopped me mid-block. I couldn't find a parking place fast enough. Finally, I pulled into an alley and ran back two blocks to find my beautiful Indian brave. When I finally found him I was out of breath and somewhat at a loss for words. How do you tell an Indian he's pretty? Better come up with something better than that . . . Gee, you got a nice back . . .? That wouldn't do either. Maybe I should just forget it. Probably get a parking ticket anyway. No! That's what I'm here for!

"Hi." (Should it have been "How"? About those languages. . .)

Tom looked down at me in a side-glance of disbelief. I was wearing shorts and tennis shoes with no socks, and carrying a camera, note pad, and pencil. He looked at me again and said, "You from candid camera?"

That broke the ice. I told him at length about my interest in the Indian cradleboard. He immediately started telling of the modernization of the reservation and how most of his people were "Americanized" now.

"Oh," I said, "that's too bad." Disappointment was written all over my face, and I felt as if I had been dealt a personal blow.

"What's wrong?" Tom was saying.

"I'm sorry, Tom, I guess I've been studying the cradleboard so much lately that it never dawned on me that your people would abandon it. *You* were certainly raised on one."

Tom looked quickly to his right and left as if I had disclosed a tribal secret.

"How can you tell?" he asked intently.

Well, Buddy, I thought, *you* asked for it. I gave him a five-minute oration on posture, shoulder blades, backs, facial development, everything I had learned from Stallard and more. As I spoke he began to stand up his straightest. Then he began to grin. When I slowed down he told me that there was a lot of peer pressure from the tribe as well as "outside" (government) pressure to conform to the white man's ways. I tried to encourage him to maintain the tribal child culture because of orthodontic and orthopedic reasons. Finally he confided to me that he was resisting change.

"I was raised on a cradleboard. You are right. Not only that, but all six of my children have been raised on the same one."

* * *

Santa Fe turned into Taos, turned into reservations out in the sticks. Everywhere I went I compared Indian bodies to "American" bodies. Most of the time the Indians won. Dozens turned into hundreds, turned into thousands of observations before I got to the point that I could glance and see people as Harvey saw them. I saw that he was right. What could I do about it?

While lounging with the literature one evening I ran across some studies by Glenn J. Doman and Carl H. Delacato. Here were two fellows that rocked the boats of several associations dedicated to working with retarded children. One thing in the discussion of their theory caught my eye. Naturally, it had to be the cradleboard. Dr. Doman had traveled deep into the Amazon jungle to the Zingu River Basin. (The Amazon again. Maybe I should go there.) Here he found tribes of Stone Age Indians who opened some new avenues of investigation for him. These Indians had "no written language, no art form, and only a rudimentary way of reckoning time." They have lived this way since the dawn of history. Up the hill 2,000 feet above them, another genetically similar tribe, the Incas, had developed a highly sophisticated civilization. Doman felt that proper brain and nerve development came only when a child could crawl before he walked. He felt that a system called "patterning" occurred in the brain while a child was crawling, and that this formed the basis of brain organization. Spastic muscles, lack of the ability to focus eyes, how you walk and talk, all of this he related to the crawl-before-you-walk syndrome. This bothered me. Possibly because when I was a child my dad used "crawl-before-you-walk" as a reason why I couldn't buy something I wanted.

Doman mentioned the restrictive action of clothing, playpens, papoose racks and swaddling clothes, and how they curtail the child's sensory intake. Poor old cradleboard got zinged again.

Since that time I have seen children treated with Doman and Delacato's methods and have talked with the parents of these kids. I am impressed with their sincerity and willingness to look into other concepts. I am in no position to evaluate their neurological methods and have no quarrel with them in this respect. But *my cradleboard!* Harvey says a true scientist looks at both sides equally. What are you if you slant a little? Human, Harvey says.

Well, I fussed around in the literature until I found the "Official Statement of the Archives of Physical Medicine and Rehabilitation." They were after Doman and Delacato. Wow! Really caustic comments and suggestions for further research that would probably cost a zillion dollars. But within this obviously slanted commentary *my* Indians came under observation. I was getting as possessive about Indians as about their cradleboard. Someone noticed that these Indians were farsighted. They couldn't see six inches in front of themselves, but demonstrated superb accuracy with a bow and arrow at distances over 100 yards. The archives people went on to say that "the lack of a written language in some primitive tribes is attributed to restrictions upon crawling and creeping—an exceedingly narrow and questionable view." Narrow and questionable view? Hey—someone's on *our* side. Another report told of color testing with these people. Original tests were done asking the Indians to separate colors into groups. There was a great deal of trouble with communication here, and the Indians seemed to have no concept of differences in color. Later tests revealed that these Indians divided color by *hue,* or intensity, into light, medium, and dark—*not* as we do, by color wavelength—green, blue, red. Crawl on, I thought, there's an answer somewhere.

The subject of swaddling crept in again and again. Swaddling was nearly universal in ancient times. I have found records from equator to pole dealing with swaddling practices, but it is interesting to note that even though each people has its own reason for swaddling, they all end up doing it essentially the same way.

Polish people felt that feet and sex organs were not to be touched. Feet, especially, should *never* be put in the mouth. What does a baby do when lying on his back? As those interesting looking feet wave by, what does the cribling do? Catch them. The only positive identification an infant can make is to see what something tastes like, so into the mouth the feet go. Horrors. Polish mothers swaddled their babies tightly to prevent such a calamity.

Russians look upon a baby as a strong, dangerous-to-itself person. If unattended the baby would gouge its eyes and face with its fingernails and even suck its thumb. Swaddling was the only way of protecting the infant from self-inflicted harm.

Jewish people felt that the baby was a defenseless creature that needed warming and protecting during its development. They swaddled their children loosely and with several layers of cloth to both warm and protect them from the harsh outside world.

Laplanders and Eskimos swaddle their babies in a sling fitted to their clothing. There are two very practical reasons for this. First, a baby exposed to the extreme harshness of cold would soon die. Second, it is utilitarian to swaddle it within the mother's clothing in such a fashion that the baby can be positioned on mother's back for transport, then wiggled around to the breast at feeding time.

Polynesian mothers used a hammock-sling similar to the polar people's, but it was wrapped around mother's forehead for support. This kept the infant in a fetal-type position. I questioned Dr. Fred Feiler, an orthopedic surgeon in Colorado Springs, about this transport method and asked if that would produce a hunched-forward posture. "No," was his reply. "Babies have extremely straight backs and carrying them in this fashion would produce no detrimental effects. Side bends of the spine as seen in side and tummy sleeping are the culprits in spinal development, not fetal positions."

The American Indian lifted up his newborn for inspection and exclaimed something like: "What a badly bunched up bag of bones!" (A baby's legs cannot be straightened out at birth or for several months thereafter.) They laced their kids to a cradleboard in an effort to straighten their legs.

There were several tribes that preferred to deform the head for societal reasons. This was done during the cradling months. Most notable for their deformities were the Chinooks. Chinook artistocracy took particular pride in flattening the foreheads of their kids. Shortly after birth babies were strapped to a cradleboard with another board tied down so that pressure was applied to the forehead. After living like this for one year, the pattern was pretty well established. As adults, the Chinooks were frequently called the "Flathead" Indians. (See figure 46.)

What about the modern American mother? What is her reaction to swaddling? Horrors! We can't impinge upon a child's *freedom*. He must be able to move about uninhibited.

Time for another expert. This time I consulted a Colorado Springs psychiatrist, Dr. Paul Draper (since deceased).

"What about swaddling, Paul? Will swaddled babies become inhibited and seek your services as they grow older?"

"Quite the contrary," he replied. "I think you'll find the swaddled baby a happier, more congenial, contented baby. There has been some interesting work reported on that. Why don't you . . ."

Here we go to the library again. Everyone I know remembers good books that went out of print 50 years ago. While on the track of that book I consulted with Paul's wife. She is an expert photographer, and I was having trouble getting shoulder-blade pictures that looked like shoulder blades.

"Wanetta," I said one day, "I wonder if you could help me with a problem?"

"What kind of problem?"

"Photography. I'm interested in doing some nude photography and am having trouble creating shadows."

"What specifically are you interested in photographing?"

"People's backs."

She looked at me doubtfully for a moment, then lowered her voice, took one step closer to me and whispered, "Maybe you need my husband's professional help."

Before I had a chance to find the book Dr. Draper recommended, I ran off to a postgraduate seminar that had nothing to do with Harvey Stallard's challenges. Yet one word kept coming to my mind. *Amazon, Amazon,* the word echoed back and forth between my conscious and subconscious mind. On the second morning of the seminar, breakfast was primary on my list. As I entered the restaurant, I spotted several dentists I knew sitting at a big table.

"Mind if I join you?"

"Come ahead. By the way, do you know. . ."

That's how you get acquainted. During the progress of casual conversation one fellow turned to another and said, "You guys going to the Amazon again this year?"

Amazon? Was that my imagination, or did I hear *Amazon?*

"Yes," Clyde was saying. "We'll be going in about six weeks. Going to stay for two weeks this time."

"Hey," said Bob, "you ought to talk Huggins into going with you. He is doing all kinds of blood-chemistry studies on people. How 'bout it, Huggins? Ever draw blood in the Amazon?"

I couldn't believe what I was hearing. It must be Providence. This must be a *sign* of some kind. I tried to remain cool.

"When are we going?" Perhaps that was too pushy, so I added, "Tell me what this is all about anyway."

"There are several groups of dental missionaries in our church," Clyde explained, "and every year we go to some remote area for two weeks or so and offer dental services where there are none. We went to the interior of Mexico last year."

"People really appreciate it," injected Art.

"What church do I have to belong to?" I asked.

"Doesn't matter," returned Clyde. "We have lots of people come with us. They belong to everything."

"Some don't belong to anything," Bob said with a grin.

Clyde darted him a quick glance with a duplicate grin. Must be an inside joke.

"You could take Charlie's place," Clyde continued. "There is room for four on our plane—I'm the pilot. You'd certainly be welcome. We are going to do dentistry, but you could do whatever you want. I don't know much about what you've been studying, but with Charlie's vacancy, we'd be glad to have you."

"Could I make a phone call?"

"Sure."

I called my office to see what havoc I could cause in six weeks. That big case I had the week marked off for had just rescheduled for two months later. Now I was *sure* it was Providence. "Leave the week marked off. I'm going to the Amazon." I hung up before the shock wore off. I love to do that to my staff.

"Okay, guys, I'm set. Now give me the details."

I forgot to go to the meeting. After all, this was far more important than whatever the clinician was talking about. I had a long list of special clothing, blade-type razors, water purifier pills, etc., that I would have to compact into 30 pounds. Bob got up to leave, shook my hand and said he'd tell Charlie I was taking his place. "That won't upset Charlie at all," Bob said, and everyone enjoyed a real hearty laugh. Really hearty. Too hearty.

"Why isn't Charlie going back?" I asked innocently.

"Snakes."

"Snakes?" I felt my cheeks droop. A cold feeling crept up my spine, and when it reached my neck it pulled my ears back. *I don't like snakes.*

"What about the snakes?"

"Oh, they've got big ones in the Amazon."

I could feel it already. Respiration ceased—pulse undetectable—blood pressure zero.

Now Bob was giving me the whole story about Charlie. "Last time we were in the Amazon we arrived the day the natives were making a clearing for a new village. The trees are tall, but have short roots. There was a certain kind of snake that they use to make these clearings. This one was 97 feet long. Big snakes sleep a lot, so they catch him when he's asleep and position his head in the center of the area they want cleared. Next they drive a huge stake through the snake's head and run."

"Run?"

"You bet. When that varmint wakes up he's going to be mad. The snake will thrash around for hours before it dies, and usually by that time all the trees are uprooted."

"Impressive sight," said Clyde, "that is, to everyone but Charlie."

More laughter.

I was sober. My knees were shaking. Ninety-seven-foot snake?

"What did Charlie do?" I quizzed. I know what I'd have done. I'd have learned to fly a plane real quick.

"Charlie didn't do much more than shake," Bob continued. "The natives really laughed though. Boy, when they saw the great white father shaking with fear, they were practically uncontrollable with laughter."

"Humiliated him, huh?"

"No, they loved the tooth fixer and he knew it. In fact they loved him so much that they decided to help him get over his fear of snakes."

"Now this is serious," added Clyde. "They have a method for curing most everything, and they thought they were doing him the biggest favor they possibly could in return for his generosity toward them."

"What did they do?" I asked.

"Long about four o'clock in the morning . . ." started Clyde, then he began to snicker. Bob had to continue: "The natives threw a 20-foot snake into Charlie's tent."

My heart stopped again.

"The natives felt that if you were awakened by a snake you would feel differently about them. They reckoned that Charlie's fear of leaving the tent in the jungle was greater than his fear of snakes, so he would come to grips with his snake-fear and overcome it. Good plan. Just didn't work."

"What happened?"

"Charlie came out of that tent at 80 miles an hour—I kid you not. He was moving."

"How far did he run?" I asked, wondering for an instant how far the Amazon was from the South Pole.

"Did pretty well 'till he hit that tree."

"Tree?"

"Yeah, full tilt. Broke his nose, blackened an eye, scratched up his belly pretty bad. Yep, Charlie will be glad to let you take his place on our next trip to the Amazon."

Well, the plane left without me. I don't really care *how* the Amazonians sleep their babies. I can read about it in books. Someone else's.

* * *

I finally found the book Dr. Draper recommended—*Infant Reactions to Restraint*. It was a dusty volume guarded carefully at the University of Colorado Medical School library. It took much ado to get permission to check it out, and then I could only keep it for five days. I thought it must be pretty popular. I checked the card. Last time it was checked out was February 1936.

Infant Reactions to Restraint. That title sounded like the author should cover the subject I was looking for. Actually the word *restraint* needs to be defined first. There are two types. One type prevents physical or mechanical movement; the other holds back intellectual or emoitonal output. "You do that and you don't get the car Saturday night" is an example of emotional restraint. That's different from locking someone in a closet or bandaging the hands to prevent thumb-sucking.

Just after the turn of the century a fellow named John B. Watson was doing a lot of research on restraint of children. Rage was his big thing. He found all kinds of things that would produce rage, even in small babies. "Observation seemed to show that hampering of the infants' movements is the factor apart from all training [which] brings out the movements characterized as rage." He even went so far as to say that "the reaction occurred when the hampering was by slight constraint." From 1917 to 1930 he was the hot authority on the subject and was the most quoted researcher in the field of infant behavior. He developed, restated and popularized his ideas until they became well known in the U.S. Much of his influence is apparent today in our attitudes toward infant restraint.

In 1925 Drs. M. Sherman and I. G. Sherman, in an effort to duplicate Watson's work, found "defense movements were not at all as violent or as extensive as Watson described in what he termed rage." Then Taylor, in attempting Watson's method at Ohio State, reported that he "could evoke no constant patterned responses and concluded that he merely evoked a generalized activity." In extending Watson's work, Pratt, Nelson, and Son found that when "the whole trunk was held gently and firmly [babies] would tend more to produce a struggleless submission." They even "had a quiet response from the babies."

Dr. Wayne Dennis at the University of Virginia came to the conclusion that "there can be no isolated stimulus." He states "quite definitely that restraint of movement achieved *without* the use of intense stimulation does not cause negative, i.e., rage-like reactions in the newborn." Dennis found that among Watson's methods of operation was "holding the head between the experimenter's hands so that it could not be moved, and pressing the subject's nose with the experimenter's forefingers, as well as by using strong taste-stimuli-saturated salt solution, a very bitter quinine solution, and dilute citric acid." Dennis found in continuing studies that "with pressure on the nose or with their bodies or heads immobilized, far from showing a disturbed reaction, the babies responded with a smile." He soon recognized that "this smiling was due partly to the peculiar attachment of the subjects to the experimenters."

Dr. Dennis published observations that were similar to those I have heard from people who work in hospital nurseries. They all agree with Dr. Dennis's statement that "unemotional, firm but gentle restraint produces a more relaxed baby."

Dennis feels that Watson's researchers were communicating terror to the test babies by their own attitudes. He comments freely on "absorption of emotion by reflection," and offers mob behavior as a prime example. This *reflection* can be seen in people absorbed in watching a prize fight. They frequently have both fists clenched as if they were actually in the fight.

Contrast what must have gone on in Watson's testing with Winifred de Kok's description of "the swaddling of Italian children as an entirely happy proceeding." She concludes that "the swaddling offers a comfortable support and protection to the newborn which, far from irritating, serves as a happy bridge across the abrupt birth passage and vaguely approximates the intrauterine condition until the baby is a little more ready for the world." De Kok also noted that "the papoose of the American Indian was generally *comfortably swaddled* on a cradleboard." The same was said of the Chinooks, "who greatly deformed their children's skulls with a rock or flat board for a forehead restrainer (hence the name 'Flathead' Indian)," while the cradleboard "was comfortably padded within," as shown in figure 46.

What about deforming the head? I mentioned that the Chinooks went to great extremes to flatten foreheads in the same plane as the nose. What did this do to the brain? The brain cavity was measured by archeologists and found to be of the same volume in an adult Chinook as in someone without the deformity. To the Chinooks, a heart-shaped head was a sign of aristocracy. Apaches put a block of wood at the back of the head of their babies (most often the males) in an attempt to flatten the back of the head. If side-to-side movements were prevented, the children would develop flattened heads. If the infant had free movement of the head, as seen in the Ute, Pima, Papago, Walapai and most Mexican tribes (this information courtesy of the Heard Museum in Phoenix), normal-shaped heads would form, and *no* flattening would occur. Many pediatricians in the U.S. are concerned with flattening the back of the head. Stallard was concerned about facial development. Combine the two and you get today's philosophy: *Don't sleep the baby on his back, you'll flatten the back of his head. Turn him over and mash his face.*

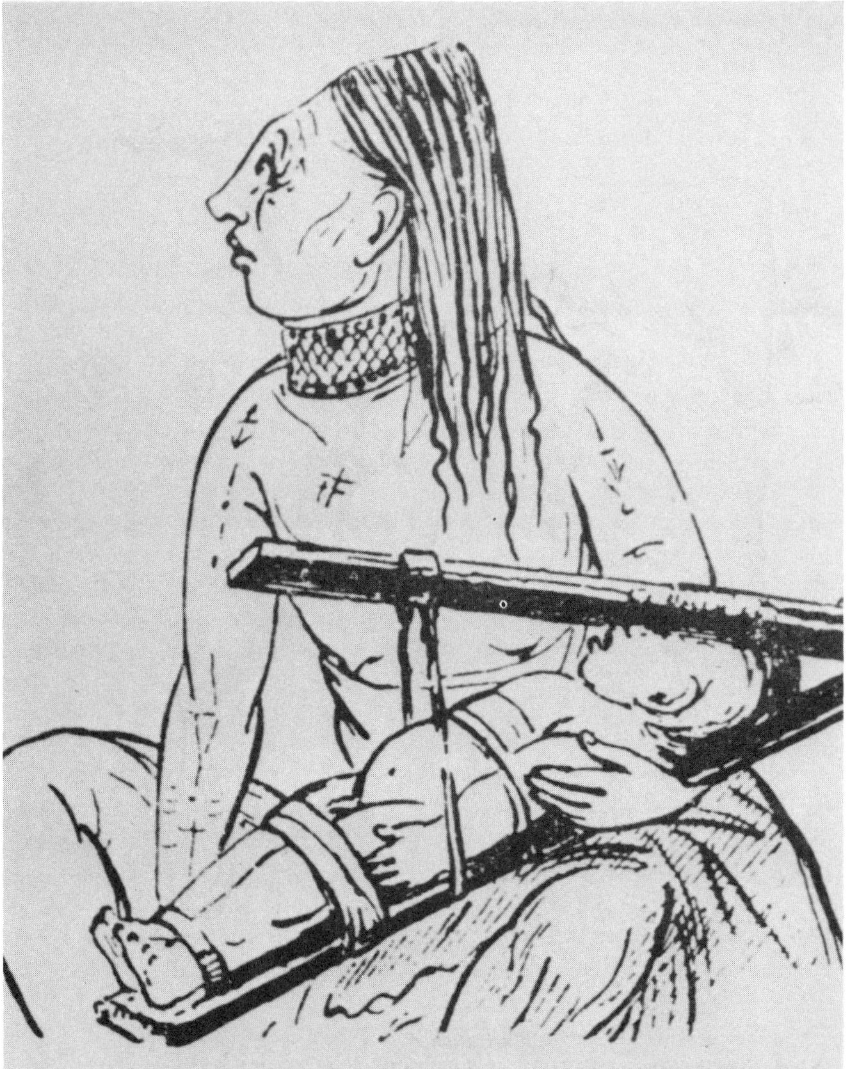

CHINOOK, from a Catlin drawing

Figure 46

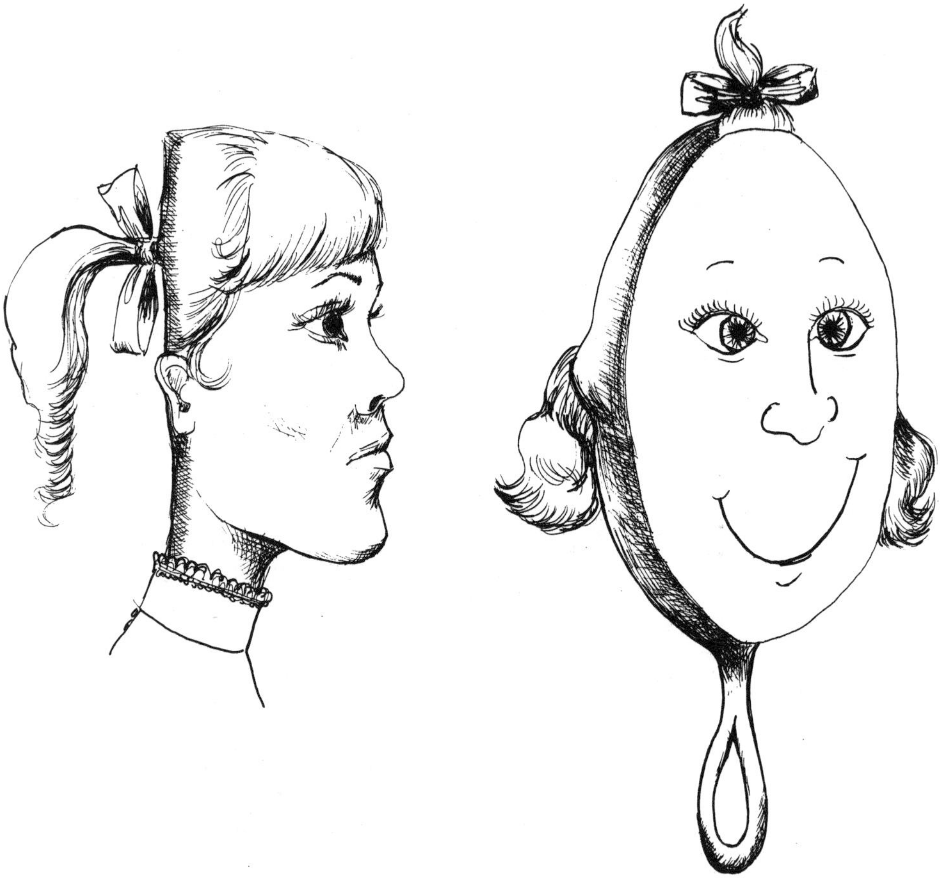

Illustration A
Don't sleep the baby on his back, you'll flatten the back of his head. Turn him over and mash his face.

Chapter Five

Why Raise Ugly Skulls?

X-rays of skulls looking face-on show the asymmetry produced by sleeping habits. This is a brand new concept and subject to many opinions. Several doctors give their views on what these skull X-rays mean.

After finishing *Why Raise Ugly Kids?* for the third time, I was relaxing from book writing by taking in a postgraduate course for fun. I didn't have to lecture one minute. I could even sleep in the back of the room if I wanted to. Dr. Karl Nishimura was lecturing on orthodontics as he saw it. I was listening with blissful complacency when all of a sudden he flashed an X-ray on the screen that hit me like a ton of bricks. It was a face-on X-ray view of a man. Usually, orthodontists take X-rays from the side of the head, not face-on. Immediately my mind went back to *Ugly Kids* and I began associating pressure to the face with this crooked nose.

"What do you think caused this?" Dr. Nishimura was asking. He'll probably say heredity, I thought to myself. Dr. Nishimura gave the audience several choices—among them, heredity. Yeah, just like I thought.

Then a most amazing thing happened. He said, "Several years ago I heard a man lecture on a subject that has completely altered my thinking on the causes of crooked teeth." The next pair of slides showed the cover of a 1971 reprint I had seen many times, "Why Raise Ugly Kids?" by Hal A. Huggins, DDS.

"I know *him,*" I said.

From the audience Dr. Roy Wolff said, "You'd better watch what you say now, 'cause Huggins is in the audience."

"Huggins, here?" said the surprised Nishimura.

"Right here," I answered.

The formality of the lecture dissolved.

"Boy, you wouldn't believe what I found after hearing you in 1973."

His rapid chatter made me feel a decade behind in two minutes. Karl had taken my work as a basis and really expanded it. He had used it in his personal and professional life. Being of Oriental descent, he still had many family ties with the old-world Oriental culture. About the time that he heard me speak on sleeping habits, his family sent him a wooden pillow from Japan. In his family's culture, if a relative gives you something, you use it. He slept on this small wooden pillow very uncomfortably for a few nights. Incidentally, the only way you can use it is by lying on your back.

"I almost cut out part of the pillow because it rubbed on one of the vertebrae on my neck. I'm glad I didn't though, because after a few days my neck changed. The wooden pillow and my neck fit perfectly. That vertebra moved. Then I became aware of the fact that my chronic neckache was gone. It had bothered me for years, but not enough to take an aspirin—just annoying. In three days it was gone and hasn't returned.

"Then I noticed another thing. I had to set the electric blanket differently when I slept on my back. I always had the blanket set on high. Within a few minutes on my back, I was too hot. I finally decided that there are more insulating fat cells on the stomach area than on the back. Ever see someone a hundred pounds overweight with a fat back? No, it all goes to the front."

Karl and I have both checked into this and find it to be consistent. There must be a lot of heat loss from the back, because both tummy and side sleepers require more covers or electric blanket heat than back sleepers. Interesting point. I found Dr. Nishimura a most brilliant lecturer.

Within a few weeks I was in his orthodontic office in Tustin, California. His highly efficient staff was very hospitable toward me, but under the smiles I could feel the "You're getting us behind schedule" daggers. My assistants are this way too. In many ways dentists are a lot like kids. When they have a new toy they like to show it to the other kids on the block.

Karl could see where a few hours of schedule interference could influence hundreds of dentists who treat thousands of patients. We both hope this is true.

Karl showed me X-rays that really demonstrated how sleeping habits play a big role in developing asymmetries in facial development. I was excited. I asked Karl if I could duplicate his X-rays. He agreed, and I decided to get "professional opinions" from doctors who would each look at X-ray pictures from a different view. Karl had given me his opinions, but he and I were obviously biased, so I gave them to doctors who knew nothing about what I was doing. What a variation. We *all* have biased opinions.

Dr. Donald Harris, a radiologist at Eisenhower Osteopathic Hospital in Colorado Springs, was the first to give an opinion. "I disagree with some of the orthodontic work," he said, "I think teeth that don't line up are pretty. I think a person with crooked teeth has that as part of his smile. It's part of his character. It's what God gave him."

In looking at the four X-rays I had selected for my opinion survey, Dr. Harris said, "I consider them all normal."

I asked him if he thought one sleeping position had advantages over another.

"An organism should sleep in any position in which he is comfortable."

I pointed out that one of his cheekbones was not developed as well as the other. "You are not symmetrical," I said.

"What difference does that make?"

"You have better development on one side than on the other."

"From the pathological standpoint," asked Dr. Harris, "how does that affect a person?"

I told him of the temporomandibular joint (jaw joint) pain that many people have. It is severe pain in those who have it, and only a few dentists in each state are competent to correct the problem.

"I'd rather say I don't understand what you are talking about. Many people in overlapping professions don't look at the same film the same way. I'd be interested in how someone's father looked, and grandfather, and great-grandfather."

"Then the tendency for these discrepancies would be hereditary in your opinion?"

"If you are telling me there is no history of trauma or disease—yes."

* * *

"The neck is where I see problems." This was Dr. Lyle Graham speaking. He is an osteopath in private practice.

"How's that?" I asked.

"If a person sleeps with his head turned to the left, there will be a structural change on the right."

"What do you mean by a structural change?"

"When the head is turned during sleeping, stomach sleeping in particular, there will be an extension and stretching of the cervical muscles on the side they turn away from. Occasionally the muscles on the other side will contract. When these people get up in the morning and try to straighten out, they can have restricted muscle activity from *both* sides. The short side will be painful from contracting, and the other side painful from fatigue. Both sides are trying to compensate for the myofacial strain that results from the sleeping position. This eventually becomes chronic and results in a malalignment of the vertebrae in the neck. This is called a structural somatic problem, or an abnormal fit between the bones. It is treatable, but tends to recur. It involves the neck most of the time, but pain can be found down as low as the thoracic area [the area of the lungs and heart]."

"What do you recommend for these people?"

"Have them sleep on their backs."

"Do you have any problem getting adults to change their sleeping habits?"

"Not really."

"I do," I commented. "After age twenty-one, people I see have a lot of trouble changing."

"That's probably due to the difference in pain."

"Pain?"

"Yes. The people I see are in a lot of pain. They don't like it. I can fix them, but it just comes back. Money is another factor. It costs them money to get out of pain. If they sleep on their back there is no pain, and it saves money. I see habit-breaking as directly proportional to the amounts of pain and money."

"Can you think of anything else that would affect growth and development?" I asked.

"Sure—other structural influences. Injuries, acquired habits—like our auditor for instance. He works on books eight hours a day. While writing figures he rests his cheek on his left wrist. Not only can this move his upper left teeth and depress his left cheekbone, but it affects his back. He is short, so when he leans on his wrist his left shoulder is higher than normal. This gives him an occasional back and shoulder problem. When the pain gets severe enough, he will break the habit, but not 'til then."

"Anything else?"

"The advent of the use of a pipe." We both laughed. Dr. Graham was smoking his pipe.

"Musical instruments put abnormal pressure on the body," he went on. "The clarinet and oboe tend to push the upper front teeth forward unless the lip muscles are firm. Some occupations cause you to clench your teeth. If you are lifting something heavy you will clench. Look at the farmer who drives a tractor for hours while looking back over one shoulder, the plasterer who does ceilings several hours a day, the grease monkey who lubricates structural systems, and show the signs in bone or muscle that reflect them. You are looking at infants where there is *no* development or maturity. I think you should look at all these places *as well as* genetics."

"I am. And genetics is the name of the game," I replied. "What I want is to find out what mechanical and biochemical influences interfere with genetics. My thought is that genetics is programmed to give us beautiful kids. All we need to do is quit interfering with it."

* * *

The next person I interviewed was Dr. Arnold Miller, a radiologist. "There are two things I look for first on an X-ray film, fractures and tumors. I don't see either in any of these films. Did you take these films?"

"No, I didn't. They were taken in California."

"I will assume they were taken with the nose against the film. If the back of the head were against the film there would be some distortion of the facial bones. Looking at film number one I note that the osseous nasal septum is deviated slightly toward the right side."

That's what I was listening for. It looked to me like a compass could draw a curve all the way down the nose shown on film number one. It wasn't straight at all. The question is, how did it get that way? Dr. Miller mentioned the importance of head positioning. If the head were turned to the left or right ever so slightly, the resulting film would be asymmetrical. This type of curve was not the type that would develop from rotating the head. He measured certain areas of the skull to check for rotation and decided that the head was in good position, and there was a curve in the nasal septum. He uses a bone called falx for a mid-line guide. Film number two also showed a curve in the nasal septum bone, which runs down the center of the nose.

Film number three showed a curve in the nasal septum, but it was different from the other two. Where numbers one and two had a curve the *full length* of the septum, number three had it only in the lower half. To me that suggested that the hand position during sleep was half an inch lower for patient number three compared to the other two. Dr. Nishimura had suggested this too.

"Look at this," Dr. Miller said. "Her eyes are not at the same level."

"Do you think the pressure during sleeping could have caused that?"

"Sure. A little gentle pressure over a period of time will really move bone. Look at the nostrils. The right one is actually larger than the left."

This went along with what I had seen looking at people's noses. "In dentistry we have an opportunity to look at noses from the bottom," I said, "and frequently we see one nostril half the size of the other."

"I never looked at noses that way," said Dr. Miller, "but I think I *will* just to see what you are talking about."

We stared at the film for a while longer, then he said, "You have me conscious of asymmetries now, and there are a lot of them between the orbits [bony sockets housing the eyes]. No particular comment—no pathology [disease] involved—just lots of asymmetry."

Looking at film number four it was obvious that the whole nasal septum was curved. The right malar process (cheekbone) was far more prominent than the left too. To me this would indicate that a hand, pillow, arm—some object applying pressure—was positioned higher than the previous patient's. Not only was the nose moved over slightly, but the pressure had prevented the full development of the cheekbone on the left side. It is hard for me to believe that heredity would build one cheek and not the other, but how about pressure preventing heredity from working? Yes, that I could see.

Dr. Miller also pointed out that the ethmoid sinus on film number four was smaller on one side than on the other.

"Look at falx," said Dr. Miller. This is that little bone inside the skull that is used as a mid-line reference point. Even falx was bent in the same arc that would include the nasal septum deviation.

Next, Dr. Miller opened a tall, skinny closet door and pulled out a skeleton. He removed the top of the skeleton's head and pointed out the bony structures we had been observing on the X-rays. Then he pointed out one thing that was the most significant bit of news he gave me.

"See this?" he asked.

"This little groove?"

"Yes. Do you know what made that groove?"

"Looks like a blood vessel to me."

"Yes."

Then what he was saying dawned on me, and he continued, "If the force of a little blood running through a vessel a little heavier than a piece of spaghetti can displace bone, then you have an idea of how easily several hours a night of improper pressures of sleeping could alter the direction that bone will grow."

* * *

Next on my list was a rare breed of professor, Dr. J. Michael Hoffman, professor of anthropology at Colorado College. He has an MD degree as well as a PhD in anthropology. My idea of selecting people who have different views on reading X-rays had wider limits than I expected. Dr. Hoffman prefaced his comments in a fashion similar to that of everyone else who had viewed the films.

"Perfect symmetry you will never find anywhere in the body."

I asked, "Is the body better off if it is symmetrical?"

"Not necessarily. It partly depends on function."

"How about if one leg is shorter than the other?" I asked.

"It depends on how the individual adapts to it."

"So, if one leg is three inches shorter than the other, adaptability would be the key?"

"Well, no, that's an obvious problem."

I decided I should lay out my ideas so he might know where I was coming from.

"I'm basing my hypothesis," I started, "on what I learned being around horses. In animal shows—horse, cow, dog, etc.—the judges look for the size and shape of the animal. This is called 'conformation.' They have learned that if an animal has a certain optimum body conformation, the functional part of the animal will also be optimum. 'Form and function go hand in hand' is a frequent statement at animal shows."

After taking this in, Dr. Hoffman laid down a ground rule I'd heard before. "We assume that the films are taken with the head properly aligned. One good check on this is to look at the nasal septum. If the nasal septum and the lateral walls of the nasal cavity are crisp, you are pretty well assured that the film and head were lined up properly. A slight rotation of the head will make the nasal septum appear fuzzy."

In looking at film number one, a tracing of which is shown here as figure 47, Dr. Hoffman said, "The first thing that hits me is the difference in the temporal vault itself. That's the skull just above the ears. The right side has a markedly smoother contour than the left. The left side looks somewhat compressed and more bumpy in appearance. Crista galli [the little bump shown in the interpretation sketch] is in the mid-line, but the perpendicular plate of the ethmoid is deviated to the right. The deviation continues down through the vomer, so the whole nasal septum is deflected to the right."

Refer to figure 47 for the positions of these skeletal structures if you're interested in detail; otherwise, here is my interpretation of what Dr. Hoffman said: Crista galli is the fairly stable piece of bone that is often used as a reference point for the middle of the head, looking face-on. The center of the nose has a bony structure called the nasal septum. It has a top half and bottom half. The top is called the ethmoid, and the bottom is the vomer. In X-ray films we sometimes see one bent, sometimes the other, but in this film, both are bent to the right from the mid-line.

Dr. Hoffman continued, "The left and right nasal cavities differ in appearance. It is hard to describe, but the lateral borders significantly differ from each other."

This means that the outer contours of the nasal cavity differ on each side.

"Another thing that is apparent," he continued, "is the total displacement of the maxilla [upper jaw] to the right. I checked the nasal bones to make sure that this is a straight-on view, and it passes. The maxilla is definitely moved to the right."

"This could be caused by having an arm under the head while sleeping," I suggested. "If the arm were over the head so that the left eye would rest on the arm, pressure would be on both the nose and upper jaw."

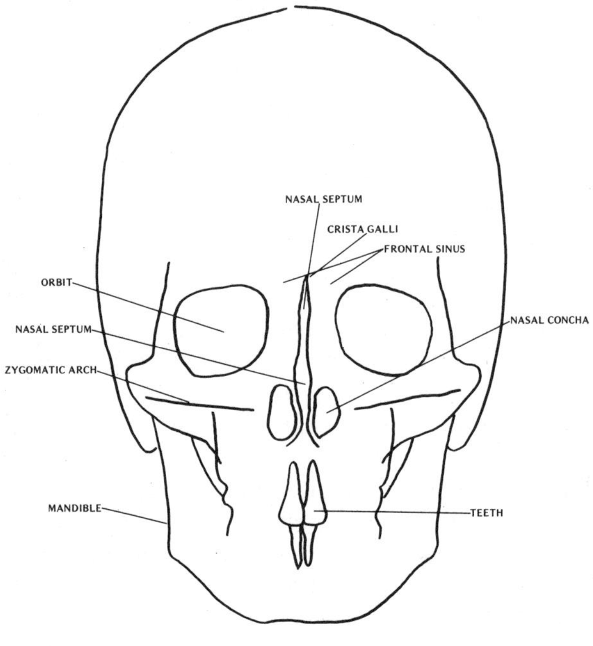

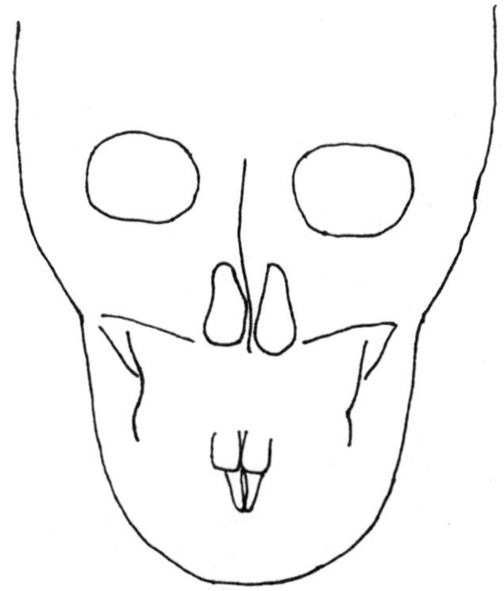

Figure 47

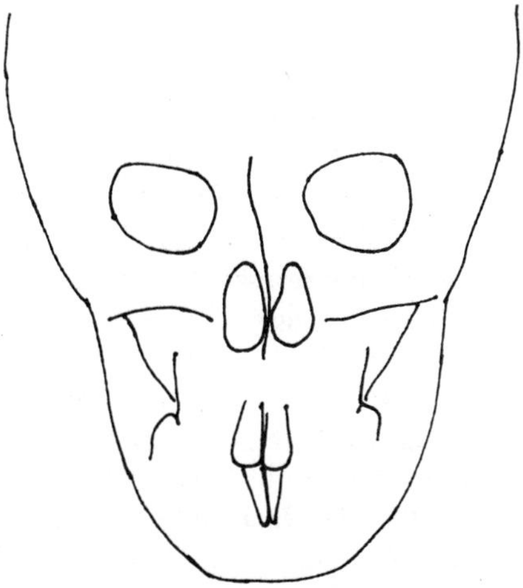

Figure 48

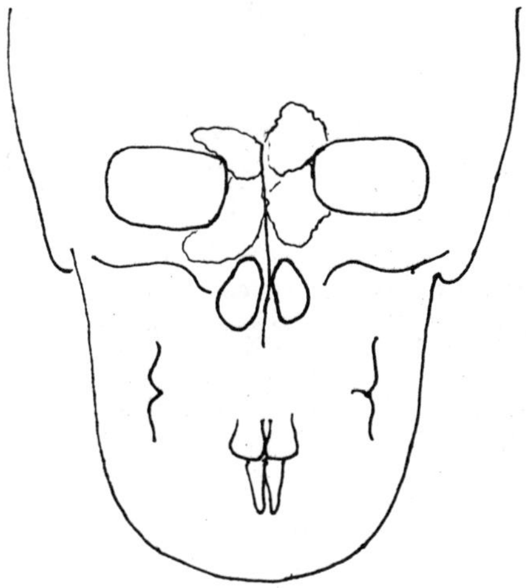

Figure 49

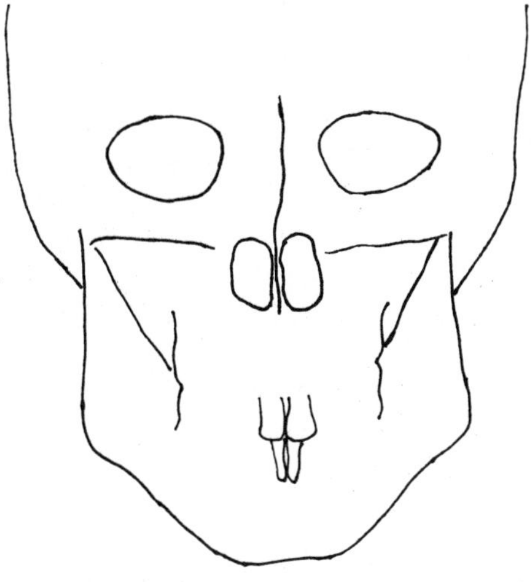

Figure 50

"Yes," he answered, "that might explain the total displacement of the middle of the face over to one side."

In looking at film number two (figure 48), Dr. Hoffman found, "It appears that the whole mid-face portion is moved to the right. This is in addition to the vomer displacement to the right. Even the bony septum that divides the frontal sinuses is deflected. The right nasal cavity is wider than the left. Also, it has a broader, flatter base. The lateral borders of the nasal cavities appear different. The right side has rounded convex borders as one would expect, while the left border is concave—just the opposite. I'll have to admit that it does look like some external pressure played a role in that type of development. Another thing that is interesting is the difference in the amount of bone around these nasal sinuses. There is far more bone around the left lateral border than the right. The right is what I would expect. The left is several millimeters thicker. The last thing I see that is noteworthy is the difference between the two sides of the chin. The right side has more development than the left."

Turning his attention to film number three (figure 49), Dr. Hoffman commented, "There are some rather obvious asymmetries here."

"Yes," I retorted, anxious to try out my newly acquired abilities at diagnosing X-rays. "That right eye is lower than the left."

"Oh?" he replied. "My impression is that the left one is higher."

"What's the difference?"

"In reference to the rest of the head, I would say that the left eye is higher than it should be."

"Displaced upward?"

"Well, yes. If you consider the whole film, it is conceivable that pressure here [at the area of the left cheekbone] could have pushed the nose and associated structures out of position. The left eye is more circular, and the right eye is more rectangular. I'm not sure what it means, but I think I'm going to be looking at films differently from now on."

I pointed out the difference between the frontal sinuses, asking, "Is this of any significance?".

"No, not really. If I were to see really symmetrical frontal sinuses I would wonder at it. They are as different as fingerprints. In fact, I know of one case personally where a dead man was positively identified by the unique shape of his frontal sinuses. We are all unique in that respect. I don't think that even the 'perfect environment' you are seeking would produce symmetrical frontal sinuses. Many of these asymmetries might not occur, but the frontal sinuses evidently have something else that controls their development."

Dr. Hoffman looked next to the nose area. "Even crista galli appears to be deviated to the left of the mid-line. The nasal septum is reasonably straight from crista down for a centimeter or so; then you can see a deviation of the vomer. I also notice that there is a big difference in the size of the ethmoid sinuses. The left one is much more compressed than the right one. The nasal cavities show the same pattern of asymmetry. In fact the length of the naris is longer on the right side than on the left side. Again, you seldom see symmetry of the nose, but this is more notable than most.

"Film number four [figure 50] shows a lot of deviation in the nasal area. There is more involvement in the perpendicular plate of the ethmoid. Note that falx is deflected, even though it is surrounded by thick bone. Something we haven't seen this pronounced is the difference in the left and right zygomatic processes [cheekbones]. The profile of the left side of the face as compared with the right indicates a possibility of pressure to that part of the face. There is a pronounced difference in the shapes of the orbits. The left one looks laterally compressed. The right one is more rounded. Left is more irregular."

He looked at me and said, "It keeps coming to my mind to ask you if you have considered the relative importance of dietary factors?"

"Yes, I am aware of the importance of nutrition, but how does it relate to your training?"

"I didn't have much in medical school—two hours talking to a nutritionist—but in physical anthropology it is a fairly well documented area."

"Are you implying that skulls and bone differ with different diets?" I felt that I was baiting him.

"Absolutely."

That took the guesswork out of my curiosity as to his feeling about nutrition, growth and development.

He continued: "Those tribes that were nomadic for centuries, then became seminomadic, on to sedentary, showed physical changes in their bodies. As nomads they subsisted on what they hunted or gathered. This was a relatively high-protein, high-animal-fat, low-carbohydrate diet. As they changed over a period of one to two hundred years (in some instances much longer) we have those skeletons to study as well as the sedentary descendants of today. In North and South America, horticulture centered around maize, or corn. As this happened, we can see a transition toward people becoming smaller in all dimensions—arms, legs, shoulders, even the teeth were smaller."

"Do you mean shorter teeth, or smaller crown size?" I interrupted.

"Both," he answered. "But not as much reduction in tooth size as in the rest of the body size. I don't know, but this could compound your problem of crowded teeth."

"Why do you think this reduction in size took place, Doctor?"

"One reason is the lack of adequate protein. Another reason is that people began to process their food. It doesn't seem to make any difference what their basic diet was; when they began to refine the foods there was less growth. This could mean using white flour or just adding sugar to the diet."

"Sounds like Weston Price," I commented.

"Yes, it does. Another factor may be of importance, and that is that refined foods require less chewing. The softer foods, combined with more refinement and a tremendous reduction of protein, resulted in people of smaller skeletal and dental development. Skeletally, we are really talking about two different things. One is the *amount* of bone—like the thickness of the cortex [outer layer] of a femur [leg bone]. The other is *density*. The nomad populations had more heavily mineralized bone as well."

"Dr. Stallard has pointed out that the diets of the ancients were high in fruits, berries, nuts and vegetables when they could get them, and that the meats were raw. Raw meat is not nearly as tough as well-done meat."

"I realize the truth to that, Hal, but I am also aware—as you are—of what happens when a tooth is removed. The bone in that area atrophies from lack of stimulation during function. Another point to be considered is that many people—Eskimos in particular—used the mouth as a third hand."

"Hand?"

"Yes! Eskimo women would chew sealskin to make it soft for footwear. The men used the mouth as a vise or as a holding apparatus to free up their hands. I don't think we can forget any of those things. They are all part of the environment that develops our bodies."

* * *

Thank you, Doctors Nishimura, Harris, Graham, Miller and Hoffman, for your views on the films. Each of you made unique comments. And a special thanks to Dr. Al Bennings, a Colorado Springs orthodontist, for supervising the skull tracings.

The consensus of opinion among the contributing physicians is that many asymmetries seen in the skull films could well have come from abnormal pressures during sleeping. Most of those asymmetries have a direct effect on producing malocclusion, so I feel it would be well worthwhile to have one of our research universities investigate the relationship between sleeping posture and skeletal abnormalities. It all boils down to the same thing, though, doesn't it? If you put pressure on thin bones, they will move. And when they do, it produces an Ugly Kid.

Chapter Six

Bending the Tooth Twig

"As the twig is bent, so grows the tree." What do we actually do to create the various types of crooked teeth?

Soon it came time to pull all my material together and make something practical out of it. My office staff was willing to work with me on the project, so we decided to make a game out of it. We all looked at faces, cheeks, posture, etc., and tried to guess what the child's sleeping position was during development and what type of orthodontic problems we would find in the mouth. I knew we were just scratching the surface, but was anxious to see a practical application of our findings. Here is the information we used as a guideline:

Observation	*Relation to Mouth*	*Probable Dominant Sleeping Position*
Good posture.	Esthetic teeth	Back
Flat shoulder blades (smooth back)	Esthetic teeth	Back
Well-developed lower third of the face	Esthetic teeth	Back
Well-developed cheeks on both sides	Esthetic teeth	Back

Observation	*Relation to Mouth*	*Probable Dominant Sleeping Position*
Straight nose	Esthetic teeth	Back
Nostrils same size	Esthetic teeth	Back
Right angle from chin to infraorbital notch	Esthetic teeth	Back
Symmetrical head shape	Esthetic teeth	Back
Head set squarely over torso	Esthetic teeth	Back
Feet "toe straight"	Esthetic teeth	Back
Stooped shoulders	Crowded teeth, especially lower front	Tummy
Lack of development of lower third of the face	Deep overbite, upper teeth hide or cover the lower when back teeth are together; high possibility of impacted wisdom teeth; possible crowding of lower	Tummy—but body chemistry plays a large role here
One cheekbone well developed, the other not	Look for crossbite on same side as underdeveloped cheek	Tummy or side with fist under face at cheek area
Both cheekbones underdeveloped	"Sad" facial appearance even when happy; look for crossbite on both sides	Tummy or side with fist under face; sleeps part on one side and part on the other
Nasal septum deviation, or crooked nose	Crossbite on the side of the face that was down	Usually side sleeping but can be tummy with hand or arm under cheek *and* nose area simultaneously
One nostril smaller than the other	Look for crossbite on small nostril side	Side, but can be tummy with hand or arm under cheek and nose simultaneously
Winged shoulder blades, both sides	Crowding generally	Usually tummy
One shoulder blade winged	Blocked out cuspid, possible crossbite in back teeth	Usually side sleeping, one side dominant
Receded chin	Excess overjet; lack of proper function; lack	Tummy

Observation	*Relation to Mouth*	*Probable Dominant Sleeping Position*
	of disclusion; crowding of lower front teeth	
Overgrowth of back of head	Usually associated with receded chin problem	Tummy
Head set forward to the long axis of the body	General crowding	Tummy
Feet "toe out" or pigeon-toed; either can occur	No definite relation to teeth other than through associated tummy sleeping problems	Tummy
Narrow face	Crowded teeth upper and lower	Tummy
Head tipped to one side	Crossbite on "downhill" side	Tummy sleeping with arm under head

The game was to make all observations by the time the child was seated in the dental chair and then talk about the dental conditions among ourselves prior to looking in the child's mouth. Usually, after three descriptive comments about the child's tooth position, his mother would speak up: "Hey, you haven't looked in his mouth yet. How can you say these things about his teeth?" You've got to get mother's attention if you're going to change anything. A comment like this meant that we had her attention.

"We did our examination on the way in. Like to see it?" Then we would let the child hop out of the dental chair and return to the door. The receptionist would stop and face the child so that my assistant and I could get a profile view while she said, "Now I'm going to introduce you to the doctor." After the introduction she would gently pat the child on the back, then hand him over to me. I would let my arm slide gently across the child's shoulders and lead him to the examining chair. As he turned to sit down I would let my hand slide down six inches on his back so that I could feel the shoulder blades as he turned to sit. Once he was in the chair we all gave him the once-over for facial symmetry. Next, I would tip the chair back—and who but your dentist gets to stare at your nose from the bottom side? The patient thinks we are looking at his teeth. Examination completed.

Of course, we would follow up with the usual oral examination, but by this time we had had an opportunity to involve *both* mother and child in the treatment of the case by creating a desire to correct bad habits. It was surprising how accurate those examinations got to be. Equally surprising was how we tended to "analyze" everyone we saw—at lunch, in the movies, at the grocery store. "Look at the shoulder blades on that tummy sleeper." "Did you see that nose?" "Man, look at that beautiful back."

Not only did we analyze the world, but we began to kid each other about our deformities. I took the prize. I was a tummy sleeper as a child (now reformed) and have the typical "wings" for shoulder blades. It is generally accepted around the office that if I were caught in a 15-mile-an-hour wind, I could fly.

Chapter Seven

Why Lose Face?

Much of the development of the lower third of the face is diet dependent. Facial growth blueprints require certain raw materials. Without them, we lose parts of our teeth, jaws, chins, and beauty.

Up to this point I had been studying the mechanical aspects of Ugly Kids. Strictly pressures and positions. Harvey had made continuous references to Dr. Weston Price and his work with nutrition. Both of these men recognized a biochemical-nutritional cause behind improper development. I felt it was time to bounce down the next set of rapids, and so began a more intense study of Weston Price's book, *Nutrition and Physical Degeneration.*

Leafing through the book as I customarily do—from back to front—I was stopped by a comment on page 514: "One of the most serious of the present confusions is failure to appreciate that an adequate, well-balanced diet is capable of building people strong and well in all respects and adequate for maintaining health and strength." Yes, there is a lot of confusion regarding nutrition.

I continued to leaf until I found a section on the use of a butter concentrate to increase mineral absorption. "In the movement of teeth consideration of mineral metabolism should be prime." I continued. Price had found that rampant dental decay (gobs) could be controlled by changing diets. During the Depression, Price was working with a Southern mission that seemed to have a never-ending supply of sick kids with lots of decay. He showed by blood tests that, as butter was increased in the diet, blood levels of calcium and inorganic phosphorous improved. Then he showed further improvement when sugar and white flour were removed from the diet and replaced with honey and whole grains. This was just the tip of the proverbial iceberg compared to what we have now found in diets that alter the blood picture. Many thanks to Weston Price for opening the door to more secrets of how to avoid raising Ugly Kids.

Price suggested that the dental arches failed to attain their full genetic development when certain fats were missing. He developed a chemical test that measured a substance in butter that was associated with resistance to decay and stimulation of bone growth. Chemical tests were not as specific then as they are today, therefore he was not exactly sure what he was measuring. The substance had some of the characteristics of vitamin A and the four D vitamins, but tended to go up in concentration as vitamin A went down. He noted the lateral incisor (number two from the mid-line) was set in toward the palate and the cuspid more outward into the lip when these fatty substances were low in the diet.

We applied this tidbit in the office, again by playing guessing games during the initial examination. I would muster up my best matter-of-fact expression, turn to mother and ask, "Why did you raise him on margarine instead of butter?" Attention getting. We counted over 100 cases and *never* missed. That seemed incredible. In every case we checked, if the kid was raised on butter, his facial form and tooth position were markedly better than those raised on margarine, *regardless* of sleeping habits. Another variable diagnostic tool was added to our list. I gradually got more and more mothers to switch to butter and thought I could see better results.

Realizing that I would be biased, I related this information to several other men who practiced orthodontics. Within three months they all told me of slow-moving cases that suddenly responded better. This was especially true of patients wearing removable orthodontic appliances. An orthodontist can't get the positive pressure with removable appliances that he can with bands that are cemented to the teeth.

I was really suspicious of this observation for several years, then heard so much from colleagues that I began to use it as part of the original consultation in the following manner. "Okay, Mrs. Mother, Johnny's orthodontics will come to $800. Oh, are you going to keep him on margarine?" If the answer was yes, I would turn to my assistant and say, "I'm sorry, would you please add $300 to the estimate?"

"Add three hundred dollars?!" I had her attention.

"Yes, teeth move much slower when the child eats margarine instead of butter. The difference is in time and millimeters, and those two items equal dollars spent. If you have the money to waste, I have the time for longer treatment."

Once in a while a mother would push for an answer as to *why* butter activated bone metabolism. In such cases, I was really stuck, because it just hadn't been investigated that much. It wasn't until 1976, when I read Dr. Daphne Roe's *Drug-Induced Nutritional Deficiencies,* that I began to understand what was happening. Roe was the first author I found who mentioned the gastrointestinal tract as a fat-soluble membrane. What that means is that nutrients will be absorbed better from the intestines if they are combined with fats.

This explained what Price had seen in Africa. He noted that people in central Africa who adopt the white man's sugar and refined-flour diet while limiting their fat intake have narrow nostrils and a marked lack of development of the lower third of the face. This refers to a smaller chin and a narrowing of the lower jaw. Crooked teeth in the lower jaw would naturally be expected. If growth was interrupted more, it was evidenced by a lack of development in the middle third of the face as well. This would mean underdevelopment in the areas of the cheekbones, roof of the mouth, upper teeth, nose, ears, and possibly eyes. Orthodontically speaking, this lack of development leads to what is called the deep overbite. *Deep overbite* is a term used to describe a situation where the upper front teeth completely hide the lower front teeth when the back teeth are closed together. How would this underdevelopment of the jaws affect wisdom teeth? Right. Impacted. Whoopee! (Negative enthusiasm to be used with this exclamation.) Price found that people are people. After identifying the causes of these underdevelopments in Africa, he found them everywhere.

At the opposite weather extreme from Africa, Price interviewed a physician who practiced in Point Barrow, Alaska. This doctor found that over a 30-year period young women in his practice were having far more complications with childbirth than their mothers had experienced. In fact, during the first few years of his practice he *never* saw a birth. It was not that the people were shy, but that birth was rapid and not complicated. The last years of his practice produced many obstetrical-gynecological problems. Long labor was common. Breech births and Caesarian sections were no longer rare.

During Price's interview with this doctor, one thing became evident. There had been a change in physical structure. Women had pelvis structures that were narrower than their mothers'. Men had changed also.

They had narrow shoulders as compared to their fathers. *Both* sexes had narrow palates in their mouths, and many of these afflicted people had crowded teeth. The lower third of the face had *not* developed properly.

Why the change in structure? Price found the same thing he had seen in other countries. There was a reduction in fats and an increase in white flour. In a film recently produced by the Price-Pottenger Foundation, there is a section of an original movie of Weston Price himself. He says, "I come to you as a missionary from them [the primitive people he studied] to the people of modern civilization, and I beg of you to learn of their accumulative wisdom. And if you do, you too can have strong healthy bodies without so much disease as we suffer from these days." Price felt that physical degeneration came from the same place the world over: "foods of commerce."

Adding one more factor, Price mentioned premature aging. He was not talking about people in their seventies or eighties, but premature aging in young people. The two sisters shown in figure 51 are a good

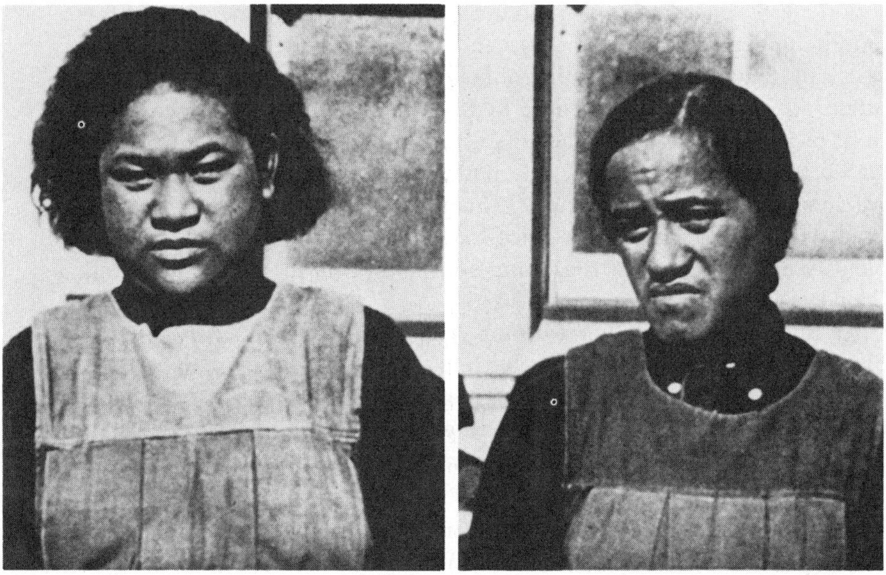

Figure 51

example of what foods of commerce can do. The sister on the right is the *older* sister. Shocking, isn't it? Note that the facial forms we have been talking about are present. Lack of development in the cheeks, lack of development in the lower one-third of the face—and marked aging.

And here again we have the same old causes—lack of fats in the diet for adequate absorption and the addition of white sugar and white flour. Price's work on physical degeneration extended beyond the mouth, but lack of development in the mouth was to him a sure sign that there was interference in the whole genetic pattern of the body.

* * *

I wondered if anyone else had noticed a correlation between development in the mouth and development in other parts of the body. It didn't take me long to find out.

One morning when I was headed for a breakfast meeting I happened to run into Dr. Frederick Feiler, a local orthopedic surgeon. Feeling a little devilish I said, "Hey, Fred, you're not going to believe this, but I can look at a person's mouth and tell you what shape his spine is in."

"Hey, Hal," he replied, "you're not going to believe this, but I can look at a person's spine and tell you what shape his mouth is in."

"No kidding?"

"Sure, we're just looking at two ends of the same elephant."

We met later that week and had a really enlightening discussion.

"There is a type of idiopathic scoliosis," Fred was saying, "that is a very distinct condition. It is a form of curvature of the spine." *Idiopathic* means we don't know what causes it. It occurs in girls a lot more often than boys and is generally noticed more during the last growth spurt. It is associated almost universally with a malocclusion—sometimes an open bite, sometimes a closed bite, a narrow arch and high palatal arch (roof of mouth). A lot has been published from the University of Illinois on the correlation between the spinal condition and improper mouth development. Narrow arch, high palate, scoliosis. (Could this be a combination of sleeping habits and the factor Price was looking for in butter?) I told Fred about the gal in Phoenix who was studying "congenital hip dysplasia."

"I don't think all hip dysplasia is congenital. Some of it is, definitely. It can be described at birth. I think one also finds hip dislocation. This can occur after birth. I think what you are talking about is a developmental problem—yes—but it occurs during early development after birth." Then he went into an elaborate description of measuring bones and angles of bones involved in the hip. He used the term *acetabular index*.

This is a measurement of the angle at which the leg bone goes into the hip girdle.

"If the acetabular index is less than 35 degrees, things should develop okay. Take an index of 25 degrees, for instance—there's no way that hip is going to let the leg become displaced. If the index is greater than 35 degrees, that is steep, and the head of the femur [top of the leg bone] can ride out of the hip joint. There is a bony lip that forms on the pelvic girdle and it helps keep the leg bone in place. It begins to develop during the first few months of life."

"What can you do with a child who has an acetabular index greater than 35 degrees?"

"Double or triple diaper him. Hold those legs apart."

I thought of a picture a missionary had given me the year before. "Then those African mothers who carry their babies by letting them straddle their hips have the right idea?"

"Yes. Africans and Eskimos both produce kids with great backs and legs, but carrying a child in that fashion usually tears *mother* apart. I see mothers in *this* country who carry their kids on a hip—not always straddled, but supermarket style I call it—and they create awful problems in their own backs.

"I think that heredity does play some role here, though, because there is an isolated area in Sweden where if a girl doesn't have a limp from a dislocated hip everyone thinks there is something wrong with her. Another classic example of heredity is found in the German shepherd dog. They have been inbred so long that congenital hips are a real problem."

Later, I recalled this part of the conversation in conjunction with something Tom (the New Mexico Indian) had said. He talked about the melding of cradleboard ideas, with many tribes borrowing ideas from other tribal designs. He spoke of the footboard on the bottom of the Hopi cradleboards and told how some Apaches used it but that the Apaches pulled the string through the footboard so tightly that it put pressure on the legs. Tom had frowned when he said that. I had forgotten it. Could it be that if you had a child with an acetabular index of close to 35 degrees and bound the legs close *together*—just the *opposite* of Feiler's preventive treatment—then added a bit of pressure from the foot end, you just might *create* a "congenitally" displaced hip? All of a sudden a complex problem dissolved into a simple solution. Here again man is *creating* a problem, then blaming it on heredity to give himself absolution.

Another spinal disease Feiler pointed out was Scheuermann's disease. This is seen primarily in adolescents and it is attributed to a growth disturbance on the anterior (front) part of the vertebral bodies, so that instead of growing as rectangles (looking from the side) they grow as wedges. Pile a bunch of wedges on top of each other and you have a curve. The flat scapula (shoulder blade) cannot fit on a curve; as a result, you have a winging of the scapulas. I have wondered what makes these vertebral bodies (building blocks of the spinal column) grow like wedges. Isn't it possible that the tree grows as the twig is bent? This whole development problem could have a relatively simple answer. I understand now the challenges Stallard faced and see why it may take years before modern research looks to something as simple as sleeping habits when it already has explanations—even if they are idiopathic (of unknown origin).

"What do you feel is the best way to sleep, Fred?"

"On your back."

"Is that a fairly uniform concept shared by orthopedists?"

"Yes, I believe it is. In fact, if you want my opinion on the *best* way, I would say on your back with a pillow under your knees. If you lie flat on your back on a flat surface, then there will be an increased arch in the lower back. This is not good."

I thought that sounded pretty uncomfortable—wrestling with an extra pillow all night. I thought that until I pulled my back out of place. Then I found how easy it was to sleep on one's back with a pillow under the knees. That was the *only* position in which I was free of pain. Another attention getter!

"What about side sleeping?" I asked.

He hesitated a moment. "Not *too* bad, if you sleep with one leg drawn up—the top one generally—and if you have a good bed. Many mattresses sold today—even the high-priced ones—are given the label 'good bed.' I find most of them are too soft. Here's what happens if you side sleep on a soft bed." He sketched a picture of a curved spine. I picked up a pencil.

"Here's what happens during side sleeping from the dental standpoint." I sketched in hands under the face. We both agreed that side sleeping produced problems.

"What about tummy sleeping?"

"That's the worst of all. You are putting three curves into the back simultaneously. First of all, the head has to turn. With a baby's minimal muscular development his head turns farther than an adult's would turn. This produces a spinal twist, which is verboten." (German for *forbidden.* Feiler is German and knows about 50,000 words of the language; I'm part German and know 16 words, so we discuss things in German as vocabulary permits.) "The rump is usually stuck up in the air, producing another curve in the back, and since the head is turned to one side, there will be a compensating curve sideways in the back, produced by the back muscles. The feet would be turned even more than the sketch indicates. This compounds tibial torsion."

"What's tibial torsion?"

"You remember from comparative anatomy that ontogeny recapitulates phylogeny?"

"You had the same instructor I had? I thought he made up those terms."

Basically, this all has to do with the study of comparative anatomy. Here you cut up a frog and draw pictures of his heart, muscles, nerves, etc., then take a pig and do the same. Then compare anatomies. There is a lot of similarity in mammal development, but the whole story can be seen by watching development from fertilization on. As a human being develops from one cell to a baby at birth, it goes through the stages of development that Darwin described. During one of the last stages—the reptilian stage—our legs are developed for reptile-type walking. As we humanize and become upright there is the tendency in the legs for reptile-type walking. When a reptile walks, his knees face out and his ankles face forward. His feet and thighs are 90 degrees to each other. As we convert to walking upright, we rotate our tibia 90 degrees; our feet and thighs face the same direction. This twisting is called *torque.* Since it registers in that part of the leg called the *tibia,* it is called *tibial torsion.* If this is not corrected naturally, it results in a condition known as pigeon-toedness. It is quite noticeable in a child when sitting with his feet dangling. Correction for this condition is done by wearing a "Dennis Brown" splint (a bar with shoes on it), which essentially holds the feet in a position similar to that found in back sleeping. When a baby sleeps on its tummy, the feet can turn in easily. When this occurs, it forces the feet into a pigeon-toed position and keeps them there. Back sleeping allows the feet to turn outward during sleep and permits natural derotation of the tibia for proper human walking.

"I'm recommending a lot of waterbeds now," said Fred. "They solve many problems simultaneously. First, there is good support of the back, second, you don't need a pillow, and last, it's easy to sleep on your back."

Another comment I might insert here is one from a specialist in pediatrics. He told me that babies are *belly breathers* and that proper breathing *cannot* be accomplished if a baby is flat on its stomach. That's why they hike their hind-ends up in the air. It's not cute; it's survival.

Feiler mentioned a theory suggested to him by an orthopedic surgeon at the Air Force Academy. The Air Force doctor felt that if people moved frequently during sleep there wouldn't be any pressure anywhere long enough to do any noticeable damage. That sounded pretty sensible, but when I mentioned it to Stallard, he said that uncomfortable people move frequently. If the bedroom is too hot, fitful sleep will result. If the internal organs become cramped, a person will move to another position.

That sounded pretty sensible too, but it brought to a head a problem I had already run into. How can you find out how people sleep and how long they stay in one position? I knew one thing for sure: *People don't know how they sleep.* Ask a man or woman in the presence of the spouse. Almost always one starts with his opinion and the other interrupts with a forceful "That's not so," or "You do not." When the human factor becomes too great one must resort to machinery. I had a friend who was an electronics whiz and he designed and built "the sleeping machine that stays awake all night." A *position sensor* recorded eight different positions on a time chart so that I could identify right side, left side, back, and tummy with the capability of registering slight variations. The sensor part of the device fit in a cap so that it could be positioned at the top of the head. From this I was able to correlate posture and profile with sleeping habits. From this experiment I found that back sleepers can stay in essentially one position comfortably for up to one hour and fifteen minutes. Other positions were rarely maintained for more than 10 to 15 minutes.

"Well," said Fred, "what are you going to do, try to educate the whole medical profession to this way of thinking?"

"No, I've tried that."

"So have I."

I was surprised. "You mean you have tried to talk about back sleeping and run into brick walls?"

"Yep. What did they say to you?"

I remembered the response I had received and somehow felt better knowing that Feiler had had the same problems. "I talked to a pediatrician once about tummy sleeping in conjunction with creating orthodontic problems. His answer was, 'That's what we have orthodontists for.' I mentioned back problems and his reply—"

Feiler took the words right out of my mouth: "That's what we have orthopedic men for."

"You know," I confessed, "I can't put a mouth together orthodontically as well as Mother Nature can."

"Nor can I orthopedically."

We sat in the silence with out own thoughts for a moment, then his face lit up. "Why don't you try the OB men?"

* * *

I'm off to see the OB, the wonderful OB . . . of Denver.

"Fantastic—this is just what the gals need while waiting to deliver."

I was completely caught up with his enthusiasm. Nice guy. If I ever have a baby, I'm going to him.

"Pregnant gals are hungry," he continued. "I can't keep enough literature in the reception room. They devour it faster than we can replace it. When gals are pregnant with their first child they want to read everything they can get their hands on. This is the place to hit them with concepts. Let them digest it now when they have time. After delivery they are so hassled and busy with diapers, husband, no sleep, etc., that they can't even keep up with the comic section of the newspaper."

Well, I had found one division of the health professionals that agreed with Feiler and me. And just in the right place. What better time to get things started than before birth? I was happy.

Is there a negative viewpoint on back sleeping? Certainly. The first one I ran into is that if a baby lies on its back and spits up it will inhale its own vomitus and die. Sounds reasonable. I went to a local pathologist—the coroner in this instance—and asked about infant mortality. That's when I found out about crib deaths, or sudden infant death. Children—not wee babies, but often several months old—are found dead in their cribs. No preliminary sickness, no sounds—and awfully hard to explain on the autopsy table. At the time no one was really sure what happened in these cases. There were many theories, but no one wanted to push much farther than to call them theories. One of the women in my office went back over eight years of police records to determine what position crib-death kids were found in. All but one were on their stomachs. The one that was on its back was not a good example because its parents were both on hard drugs at the time of conception. The pathologist stated that all the internal organs were abnormal in size and in abnormal positions within the baby's body.

From here I went to the head nurses of several hospital nurseries. This is a different world from the rest of the hospital, sort of a separate kingdom. They seem to make their own rules and abide by them. I can't visualize administrative policy having much effect in this zone. In most other hospital departments there is conversation about which department got increased allocations and which gal got Christmas vacation two years in a row. This wasn't apparent in the nursery. I suppose it goes on, but the nurses have to gripe quickly. Maybe they are all vicarious little mothers of the moment and think more about their jobs. It looks like a fun place to work. A white world with eyes peering out here and there, white dresses and pants, white caps, masks, shoes, and stockings. How I hate white nurse socks. Ugly.

Somewhere in the midst of all this is King Kong. She has been head of the nursery for 30 years and runs the place with one iron hand and one made of rose petals—the iron hand for the doctors and rose petals for the kids. With all due respect, I think these head nurses merely "tolerate" doctors. "What do they know about the 24-hour child?" one head nurse with a deep voice demanded of me. "They flit in here, examine the kid and are gone for another 23 hours and 55 minutes. We have to keep them 24 hours a day."

I noticed that big mama was wrapping a baby snuggly. "Swaddling?" I asked.

"Oh, yes. The little elves get along much better in this world if they are snug as a bug in a rug."

Not quite the way the psychiatrists put it, but I think it was the same idea. I told her of my interest in child culture and made mention that many societies lay their babies on their backs.

"We do that here generally—except when the doctors are making their rounds. Some doctors are finicky about feeding the kids and laying them on their stomach. This just makes them spit up. How would you like to lie on your stomach just after a big meal?"

"Doesn't sound comfortable. Isn't that supposed to vent the gases off the stomach better though?"

"Oh, from the scientific point of view, I suppose so. If we have a problem kid, though, I just prop him on his side. But you know where the problem is, don't you?"

"Where?"

"Milk. If you feed the child his God-given first meals you don't have as much trouble as with that artificial stuff. More gals are going natural now though. Just in the last ten years I've seen a big increase in numbers. Glad to see it. Gotta run."

Milk? Looks like nutrition is cropping up again. Another frontier to investigate. Maybe mother's milk *is* better. It's certainly more economical and convenient.

I was in another hospital late one night, setting up some equipment I would need for an early morning surgical case, when I heard a baby crying. A new baby just born that afternoon was exercising its lungs to maximum capacity. I talked with the nurse on duty and asked if I could swaddle the child. She had me "mask and gown" and let me in. Now, swaddling was not my most highly developed skill, but I had watched some pros, so monkey see, monkey do. I took the bunting blanket and wrapped it snuggly with the arms against body and tucked it in. Almost immediately the child became quiet and went to sleep. Wow! It worked. It was only one case, but it was successful. Feeling quite elated with the results of my newfound, age-old wisdom, I slipped from the nursery on cloud nine. It wasn't often that I was able to ply my new trade—swaddling.

Another negative—a big one—snoring. Some people sleep on their backs and snore. That was a short-lived investigation wanting much research even today—primarily in the area of an answer. I interviewed 36 chronic noisy snorers and found one reasonably common denominator in 30 of them: tonsils. They had their tonsils removed *twice*, or had had them removed *after* age 21. What does this mean? Not much. I have found scads of people who sleep on their backs and *don't* snore, but that doesn't make headlines.

Back to the master. I asked Stallard about snoring. "Why, that's a *social* problem—has nothing to do with health."

I repeated this to a dentist's wife who was complaining about her husband's nocturnal symphony. "Does too relate to health," she replied. "If he starts that again I'm going to mash his skull."

* * *

Dr. Archie Kalokerinos, an Australian MD, has finally made a stand on sudden infant death. He practiced medicine among the aborigines in the bush country of Australia for several years and was plagued with sudden infant death. In his book *Every Second Child,* Kalokerinos describes his frustration at having kids die right under his nose—that is, under close supervision in the hospital—then his search for an answer, testing of his answer, then the personality crushing experience of fighting to gain acceptance from his medical colleagues.

Kalokerinos, or perhaps Archie is easier to say, was practicing medicine in an area that had a very high death rate for children (500 out of every 1,000—hence the title *Every Second Child*). To Archie's way of thinking, there were strange circumstances surrounding the deaths. Children would appear to be in satisfactory health, or just to have a cold, when all of a sudden they would become highly irritable, refuse food and water and then for no good reason go into shock and die. He would do autopsies on these children, sometimes within minutes of death, trying to determine the cause of death. Minor changes in the liver were all he ever found.

This at least agreed with what he saw a few days before death—a liver that was tender to the touch in these kids. One time in frustration he took one of these children to a specialist 200 miles away. That's a long trip in the area of Australia where he practiced. He took the child to a Dr. Harbison, who looked at the gums and the child's general condition, and said he thought the child had a rare case of scurvy. Within less than half an hour after a vitamin C injection was given, the child's symptoms were gone.

This was dramatic, and Archie brought this knowledge back home with him. He began to review and classify symptoms and disease progress of the children he had seen die and found that there was a pattern. It consisted of a series of minor diseases, such as colds followed by irritability and diarrhea. Then out of nowhere there was sudden collapse, shock and death. Autopsy showed only liver changes. Irritability seemed to be the real red flag. It meant that death was approaching fast. A second red flag (usually coming half an hour before death) was an arching of the back and a characteristic tipping backward of the head. This was a symptom associated with cerebral irritability (inflammation of the brain).

Archie started using 100 to 200 milligrams of vitamin C by injection and noticed that within 20 minutes the symptoms disappeared and the children would take nourishment, whereas a few minutes before they cried when forced to eat or drink. Within a few more minutes they generally calmed down and went to sleep. One injection was not the total cure, nor was vitamin C the only deficiency these children had. Several injections daily were required for two to four days before it was deemed safe to release the child. Years later a series of tests for vitamin deficiencies showed that nearly everyone tested was either very low or frankly deficient.

Over the next year Archie was elated with his discovery and decided to share this information with the rest of the Australian medical community. Infant death was one of the major problems among aborigines. Surely this would produce one of the biggest aids to infant health of the decade. Archie did not understand the "don't-rock-the-boat" syndrome characteristic of many scientific bodies. His recognition came in the form of comments like "unreasonable," "stupid" and "gone around the bend." From reading his book, I get the impression that Archie is a very sensitive person, and I am sure that he cried inside as he "let it all hang out" for the sake of dying children and then heard his contribution labeled absurd. Absurd because there were so many famous specialists working on the problem, and surely they would have found the answer long ago had it been such a simple thing as a vitamin deficiency. Archie's frustration shows in his chapter "They Refused to Listen," but fortunately only his interior has softness. He hardened his exterior personality to his peers' comments and started a one-man battle to gain acceptance for his findings.

He figured that there were three types of malnutrition: food deficiency, illness (a sick infant may not thrive even on a perfect diet), and malabsorption (not being able to properly absorb the building blocks from the intestine into the bloodstream). The latter seems familiar, doesn't it? So, vitamin C was not the only problem in Australian medicine; it happened to make the difference between survival and death in some cases, but lots of things had changed as the aboriginal became "civilized." His new civilized diet sounded much like what Dr. Weston Price described for other regions where the white man's influence changed the dinner table menu. Archie mentioned that "an alarming proportion of aborigines live on diets consisting of sugar, white bread, jam, and sausage. There is very little vitamin C in this."

As Archie's observations crystallized, one more disease-producing factor appeared on the horizon. During the second year it became apparent that sudden infant death was like any other disease picture—multicausal. That meant that there was not just one factor involved, but a symphony of discord. The common cold increased the need for vitamin C. Tests had shown that when a child had a cold he secreted very little or no vitamin C in the urine. This meant that the body was conserving it in the presence of increased need. The cold led to increased susceptibility to infection—then came the diarrhea. Diarrhea decreased the absorption of nutrients from the foods, and this led to lowered resistance. It was a matter of standard procedure to use antibiotics at this point. Antibiotics produced further intestinal irritation and further increased the diarrhea. A vicious cycle. Meanwhile *all* this was reducing the already low vitamin C level. If the diarrhea produced severe dehydration, then the child was given a glucose solution intravenously. Glucose decreases vitamin C and produces an increased need for B vitamins to metabolize ("burn") the glucose. According to blood tests that had previously been run on aboriginal children, most of them were already deficient in B vitamins. If one of these already deficient children fell into this disease sequence, he frequently went into shock.

All of this was bad enough. Then one day Archie picked up on another "hidden obvious." *Inoculations* deplete the body of vitamin C. If the medical society felt rocked by sudden infant death's relation to vitamin C, what would its reaction be to the idea that its immunization program was lowering the vitamin C level, thus precipitating the sudden infant death syndrome in an already sickly child? I imagine chills ran up and down Archie's spine when he made this flash connection. He hurriedly checked records, and much to his excitement and dismay, the facts fit. Looking at the areas where the inoculation teams traveled, he found rashes of sudden infant death in their wake. Many times deaths were reported within two days. This was easily tested by animal experiments. Some had already been run. Cause of death had been attributed to "anaphalactic shock." In rerunning these tests with vitamin C given prior to the inoculations, *no* animals died. Without vitamin C, 50 percent died of anaphalactic shock.

This news hit the medical community like a bombshell, and Archie was invited to speak on a panel that was discussing immunological problems. Maybe things would be easier this time. Oh? When the other panelists found out Archie was on the program they refused to appear, and the symposium was cancelled.

"He's a *rathog,*" said one panelist. (This is a big insult in Australia—something like a nerd, but worse.) Another panelist couldn't talk "for political reasons." One would not appear on the same platform with Archie lest people think he agreed with him. "Apparently there was violent opposition to my views," Archie wrote. Violent views, but who gets hurt? Physically hurt, or feeling hurt? This invites the question, should we keep the other researchers' feelings from being hurt or keep the children from being hurt? It's a big putdown to have someone prove you wrong. It sometimes pangs us for years. Every one of us has experienced it and probably didn't enjoy it. But how does *this* kind of hurt compare to the hurts placed upon the kids? Theirs was short-term. They died.

No one ever really told the whole story about the Cherbourg Aboriginal Mission Project. Even though the risk of smallpox was minimal in Australia, there was still an active immunization campaign carried out by this mission. During this particular campaign some infants got seriously ill, perhaps many died. Whatever the *silent* result of the immunization program, it brought about an immediate reinstatement of the symposium. Archie was asked to speak.

This reinstatement of the symposium was a big turning point in the process of opening men's minds. Immunization, as valuable as it is, must be conducted with careful consideration of the health status of the patient. If immunization does drop the vitamin C level rapidly, and if a rock-bottom level of C leads to the deaths that Archie had seen so often, then certainly a patient's vitamin C level should be respected. In light of the B vitamin deficiency found, perhaps *total* health should be considered before immunization.

Problems still exist today. Archie is not shining victorious, but he is definitely a glow in the dark sky of 500 mortalities per 1,000 babies. His viewpoints are being considered in light of new projects designed to improve the health of the aborigines. A summary of his proposal looks like this: Improve diets overall (a long process in light of the difficulty of returning to a native diet with the addiction to sugar apparent now). Control immunization campaigns. This would involve avoiding inoculations in certain cases, those where the vitamin C level is already potentially low. Those excused would be:

infants suffering from infections,
infants suffering from colds,
infants who are underweight,
infants with otitis media (ear infections), and
infants who have had repeated infections.

Routine tuberculosis vaccinations should be abandoned. The disease is virtually absent from the continent. In *all* cases a vitamin C dietary evaluation screen should be done. If a nonsymptomatic child shows a dietary suggestion of deficiency, inoculation should be avoided. Careful consideration should be made of the advantages of intramuscular antibiotic injections over the intestinal irritation produced by antibiotics taken by mouth.

Now that the big problems are hopefully on the way to the lived-happily-ever-after category, let's look at one little zinger that nips at mother's quiet moments. Remember teething? If you want to see a really Ugly Kid, try to fondle a baby who is teething. Ugly? They can be downright obnoxious. Maybe you have yet to be blessed with a child experiencing this little event, but it happened that one day Archie poked into it. Many experts deny that such a "syndrome" exists, but most general practitioners, pediatricians and mothers are aware of it. Archie had a friend whose baby was teething. The child's reactions struck a familiar note. This child's clinical features of teething were pretty much "textbook": the presence of red, swollen gums and a tendency toward ear infections, bronchitis, diarrhea and irritability. Sound familiar? The child's mother assured Archie that the child was on a good, sound European diet. The child was described as "a whining, crying infant incapable of either accepting or giving affection." Well, why not? Archie administered vitamin C by injection and waited. Within 30 minutes "there was a remarkable personality change." The patient was now a normal loving child. Vitamin C had had the same effect on this teething child that it had on the vitamin C–deficient aborigines.

Once more there was the thrill and excitement that accompanies a major discovery. But now Archie was wiser. In *his* words, "The story was too rich. It was obvious that nobody would believe me. In this last assumption I was right. Physicians have not accepted the use of vitamin C for the problems of teething."

Thank God for people like Archie who are willing to pay the price of peer abuse in order to bring good health to the people who need and want it.

Chapter Eight

Cholesterol—A Help or Hindrance?

Why does the body manufacture cholesterol? What does it make it out of? Find out how eating it helps us avoid being ugly.

In leafing through *Reader's Digest* in my customary fashion (back to front) I happened upon an ad. "Mother," the ad admonished in bold type, "Should You Worry About Your Child's Cholesterol?" I looked all over the ad and couldn't find the answer. Price, Page and Cheraskin had all mentioned the advantage of fats in the diet, while the general consensus of conversation (both professional and lay) said fats were a "no-no." Besides, fat makes you fat.

By this time I had several years of nutrition under my belt, so I decided it was time to look into the cholesterol controversy. I have lots of blood, so I decided to look at my own cholesterol and to read about it.

The field of nutritional research has been infested with dental researchers as far back as I can find materials relating to the subject. I guess it wasn't out of line for me to follow suit. Refined carbohydrates were listed in some of my readings as the real culprits in elevating cholesterol. One day I stuck to a high protein, low refined carbohydrate diet and took blood. Then I went on a relatively high carbohydrate diet and took blood. Then back again. My cholesterol jumped up 63 points with spaghetti, and on the low carbohydrate, high protein diet it went back down to 210 mg%. Since then, I have seen the blood tests of over 20,000 people. Some are patients of mine; some are other doctors, their wives and personnel who have attended body chemistry seminars I have conducted; and many are the patients of other doctors. Even after looking at thousands of chemistries, I have not found anything to change the original concepts developed on the basis of the first 100. That's consistency.

I needed direction concerning what to do with all this information. Then it came to me—in the form of a challenge. A pathologist (an MD who studies the causes of death and examines surgically removed tissues under a microscope) attended one of my seminars and afterward challenged me to prove a point. He noted that we recommended two eggs and a quarter pound of butter daily to raise low cholesterol levels. He also noted that we recommended two eggs and a quarter pound of butter daily to *lower* a *high* cholesterol. His comment was, "Physiologically, you cannot use the same treatment to raise something that you use to lower it." That's a good point. Perhaps what we are doing is *not* administering a "treatment," however, but allowing the body to optimize. Of course, there was one element he neglected to mention here. The key phrase, "in the absence of sugar." Sugar, the white stuff on the table (sucrose), seems to have the *biggest* influence on cholesterol levels. Although the control of cholesterol is not simple, it is not difficult in over 90 percent of cases. "This doesn't sound possible," the pathologist was saying, "but obviously you have something to substantiate it or you wouldn't be saying it. I'd like to see ten cases you've done that demonstrate this."

The result of this challenge is a study of 64 patients I published in the United States as "The Two Faces of Cholesterol" and in Canada as "Dentistry Butters Up Cholesterol." Pioneers in balancing body chemistry had suggested that the optimum range for cholesterol was 200 to 235 mg %. Page even suggested 222 mg % as a theoretical optimum level. I had my assistants pull the records of those with an initial *high* or *low* reading of cholesterol. This was *not* a random-sample selection but people who were selected because they were *not* in the ideal range. In these 64 patients who ate a minimum of two eggs and a quarter of a pound of butter daily (in the absence of sugar) we noted over three months that the lows were coming up and the highs were coming down. Actually, most of the change occurred the *first* month. By the third month it was evident that a line representing the rising low cholesterols and a line representing the falling high cholesterols were going to form a merger. Mathematically, this occurred at 221.18 mg%. Of course, actual chemical tests can't be run accurately in the decimal range, but from the theoretical standpoint on this 64-patient test, I can fully agree with the suggested

200—235 mg% optimum range. We still use a range of 200 to 235 mg% and have good success attaining it, while the "normal" range of 150 to 300 mg % has just been raised to 330 mg % to accommodate the many new high cholesterol counts that are occurring.

Just what is it that controls the cholesterol level? Diet has a lot to do with it. Sugar may be the *biggest* culprit, but it is *not* the only one. Caffeine and alcohol also tend to elevate cholesterol levels in most people. Coffee has been sugested as a good snack food because it has no calorics and, therefore, shouldn't affect the chemistry. Maybe the coffee doesn't but the caffeine in it sure does. Caffeine causes adverse changes in blood serum levels of calcium, phosphorous, glucose cholesterol, triglyceride and uric acid, just for starters. It is one of the primary elevators of the triglyceride level, which is far more dangerous to health than a high blood cholesterol. Further, we have recently found that one cup of coffee can raise blood pressure 25 points.

Alcohol in any form *can* elevate the cholesterol level, but to varying degrees depending upon the person. Dietary control of cholesterol is primarily in the hands of sugar, caffeine and alcohol, but once in a while a sleeper like fruit juice creeps in. That's one way we can tell if someone is drinking too much fruit juice. The cholesterol will go up. This type of dietary control of cholesterol works in more than 90 percent of the cases. In those stubborn ones that don't respond readily, usually the problem is in chromium metabolism. Our bodies use chromium as an activator of energy-producing systems and cell membrane chemistry that help keep cholesterol at its proper level. Sugar depletes the body of chromium, and if one has consumed sugar over a period of years, the cholesterol will not come under control until the chromium level is built up. This usually requires taking it in pill form for a while because few of our foods are rich in chromium anymore. Potassium is necessary in a few of the stubborn cases, and in others, both potassium and chromium are required in addition to proper diet. There are still 2 or 3 percent that do not respond well, but the success of this method is a big step ahead of drug therapy.

* * *

I kept thinking about "worrying about your child's cholesterol" in that ad. Since the body manufactures cholesterol daily, and can make it out of almost any food we eat, does cholesterol have a role to play in proper growth and development? Answers were few and far between at first, then they began to fit into place. Remember that book I mentioned, *Drug-Induced Nutritional Deficiencies,* by Daphne Roe, MD? She mentioned that the intestines are a fat soluble membrane. This means that fats are absorbed easily through the intestinal wall. Could it be that the vitamins, minerals and other "building block" forms of nutrients are absorbed better when they are *combined with* fats? After reviewing a stack of chemistry reports that suggested this would be true, I hurriedly called Dr. Joseph Rabinowitz, a renowned chemistry researcher in Philadelphia. He had written several good articles and a textbook on biochemistry. I told him of my observations and asked if he could substantiate it.

"I know what you are seeing," he said, "and lots of other people are seeing the same thing. For this reason I have been watching the literature closely and have seen lots of controversy, but no good article to say what is or is not happening. Seriously, I am 'up' on the literature, and it just isn't there."

If it is true that minerals and other nutrients are absorbed better in the presence of fats, then this might explain why Price found fewer cavities and better bone around the teeth when butter was added to the diet. It was Price who noted that cultures that included higher amounts of fat in their daily diets had lower percentages of degenerative diseases (diabetes, arthritis, cataracts, gum disease, dental decay, hardening of the arteries) in their populations. Although this conflicts with some modern thoughts, he had *lots* of evidence to support his views.

What about the saturated fats versus the unsaturated? My patients' chemistries sure looked better with *saturates* present. Did I see just a select type of people? What about other regions?

To examine this first hand, I had an interesting conversation with Dr. and Mrs. Lester Lonergan (my wife's parents). For several years they have been doing medical missionary work in Africa and in the Philippines, training natives in paramedical procedures. Dr. Lonergan had taught in a medical school for 35 years and was pretty well ingrained with the fats-are-bad philosophy. After a few years in the bush country his attitude began to change, for in most of those areas where coconut oil (high in saturated fats) was a staple of the local diet, heart disease was at a minimum. The couple found, much as Price had nearly 50 years before, that as the natives became exposed to the American diet, their teeth went first. When a man would come in from the bush for training, they would look at his mouth first. "White-man's-diet disease" was easy to spot. If he had good teeth he would probably make a good paramedic because he was still thinking the native way. If his teeth were decayed, more emphasis would have to be put on resisting the sugars that were so addicting to these people. Were fat-eating natives fat? Not generally so considering the amount of fats they ate.

Let's look at people of another area. According to Kan-Jey Ho, MD, and his associates, who study Eskimos, "as a rule Eskimos are powerfully built with relatively non-obese short and large musculo-skeletal physiques." Possibly it is their clothing that makes them look rotund.

We have seen many patients in our practice lose lots of excess weight when adding fats to the diet, possibly because excess carbohydrates are a prime factor in excess weight. Not everyone loses weight easily, and men seem to lose it more easily than women. (Taking my own case, when I first got into body chemistry, I lost over 25 pounds on a high-fat diet. I don't have all the answers to weight control, but I do know that efficiency of the body chemistry has a lot to do with it. For sure, though, fats don't seem to be as big a factor in weight gain as I once thought. Quite the contrary.

Okay, so fats are necessary for absorption of essential ingredients of cellular metabolism (energy production). What else do they do? Let's take cholesterol in particular. Cholesterol in the presence of sunshine is a primary ingredient in the formation of vitamin D. Vitamin D is needed in bones for proper growth and development. Cholesterol is the basic building block of testosterone and estrogen, the principal male and female sex hormones. Are these necessary for proper growth and development? Necessary? They are absolutely *essential!* The transition from childhood to adulthood is dependent upon adequate hormones to bring about the change. Anything else? Yes, red blood cells are composed of two membranes stuck together with "glue." What do you suppose that glue is made from? Right—cholesterol. In fact, some of the energy used for normal reactions in the red blood cells is derived from cholesterol.

Nerves are like electric wires—they conduct electrical impulses. Just as a television set could short out if bare wires touched each other, there are essential areas of our bodies where the nerves have insulation around them to prevent similar shorting out. This insulation is called the myelin sheath. What do you suppose the myelin sheath is made from? Cholesterol. I've seen conflicting figures on how much of the brain is made of cholesterol, but the minimum figure I've seen is 15 percent.

All this makes cholesterol sound like an essential ingredient in proper growth and development.

How about it, should you worry about your child's cholesterol? Yes, I suppose you should. See to it he gets plenty.

Chapter Nine

Why Eat Ugly Foods? Diet for Pregnancy and Child Development

Two generations back, the family doctor had the responsibility of instructing pregnant women in how to produce beautiful babies. Nutrition was a big part of this instruction. Everyone was closer to the farm then and it was easier to see that what you sow is what you reap. This was true for crops, farm animals, and people. Care and feeding of pregnant females was very important then. Let's look over these nutritional suggestions and see how our ancestors avoided raising Ugly Kids.

Before the advent of antibiotics, tranquilizers, jet planes and all the things that make our lifestyle fast and hectic, there was a different breed of doctor. Today we have over 200,000 drugs available to us through many large industrial drug houses. Thousands of drugstores are ready to fill the doctor's order swiftly by telephone prescription, and relief is on its way. This has not always been the case. Just a few short decades ago—with *no* antibiotics and *no* tranquilizers available (these items constitute 40 percent of today's drug market)—doctors had an entirely different method of treating patients. The days of horse and buggy are gone, just like house calls and doctors sitting all night at a patient's bedside. Lots of things from the past are gone—"transisted" into modern life or just slipped into history books. Out of the past, though, I came upon a copy of what I call the "Jarvis Papers." My thanks to Dr. Melvin Page for allowing me to copy some 20,000 pages of the study club material collected by Dr. D. C. Jarvis of Barre, Vermont.

Dr. Jarvis was the mentor of a unique study club composed of about 60 MDs and two dentists who exchanged ideas for more than 30 years. This study club was unique in that it didn't hold meetings. Most of the members never even met each other face to face. It was a correspondence study club. This explains why there are 20,000 pages of material. Everyone mailed in their ideas, and Dr. Jarvis mimeographed the meaningful messages and mailed them to the membership.

It is fascinating to peek over the shoulders of these men as they told each other of new methods they were trying. Very little of this material ever got published, but this was long before the advent of the "publish or perish" syndrome. Their primary objective was to exchange ideas of a practical nature that might help on a daily basis. They didn't discuss rare diseases found on tropical islands, just runny noses and day-to-day sickness. One area that particularly caught Jarvis's attention was pregnancy and child development. He could have written a terrific book if he had used the theme *Why Raise Ugly Kids?* I'm sure he would have liked that title. He's my kind of guy.

The only sample of his work remaining today that I know about is a book on Vermont folk medicine. He found many folk remedies that worked and applied his superior analytical abilities to finding out why. Today modern authorities scoff at him because he worked with folk medicine instead of modern drugs. His work is treated as though he had studied voodoo. That's too bad, because reading a few thousand pages of his unpublished materials showed me that he had one of the keen minds of the century.

So much for ancient history. What I really want to do is show you the ideas he had concerning raising pretty babies. It doesn't take long to tell his basic philosophy, but *explaining* it requires lots of ink. (In an associated study he got involved in the medicinal use of honey. He really got turned on by honey and wrote several articles as well as thousands of unpublished words on the subject. It is not presented here with the idea of being a cure-all, but it's about as close to it as they had in the 1920s and '30s.) It's been fun to follow the progress of Jarvis's child development theories as he gained more practical experience and got feedback from other doctors who were using his ideas on their patients. I have put it together in a final plan, but keep in mind that it took him years—literally decades—to collect all this information.

His thoughts on pregnancy boiled down to this:

Expectant mother, would you like—

(1) A baby that is strong and vigorous at birth?

(2) To be able to hold your weight within normal limits while pregnant?
(3) A short labor with a quick recovery?

(Well, who wouldn't?)

Then are you willing to—
(1) Eliminate sugar, wheat, and milk from your diet?
(2) Eat soft cheese, rye bread and cornbread?
(3) Eat at least one egg daily?
(4) Eat liver, heart or tripe twice a week?
(5) Eat two raw vegetables daily?
(6) Eat nuts frequently?
(7) Avoid citrus fruit and juices?
(8) Drink grape, apple, or cranberry juice?
(9) Take two teaspoons of honey with each meal?

Here's a list of fringe benefits from this diet (also Jarvis's way of telling whether a mother followed instructions or not):

(1) The baby will be born with so much hair that it will need a haircut the first day. The baby will maintain a heavy head of hair as he grows up if he stays on a good diet.

(2) Keep the scissors out because after the haircut the fingernails will need trimming on day one also.

(3) A well-coordinated nerve and muscle system will become evident within the first week if the child raises its head off the pillow on his own accord. This is an excellent sign for proper development of the nerves *and* muscles.

(4) Mother should have an abundant supply of milk, which will enable her to breast-feed the child if she wants to.

(5) The baby should have no trouble with digestion and elimination.

(6) Mother will observe that her baby "has good width of face as a normal baby should have." (That sounds like Price talking, doesn't it? One of Price's criteria for proper growth and development was a well-developed face. Price's dietary suggestions were very similar to Jarvis's except that he leaned harder on the inclusion of fats in the prenatal diet for proper absorption of all those nutrients.)

(7) Each jaw will be horseshoe-shaped. This will enable each tooth to appear without being crowded by other teeth.

(8) Best of all, the child will be mentally alert and bright. It will be a pleasure to see how well the child does in school.

Wow! That's *heavy*. But what's it based on? It is the result of observations during *many* years of practice. It was the *parents* of children raised under these conditions who pointed a lot of this out to Jarvis. Parents would comment about how much better a child performed when produced the Jarvis way, as compared to their other children. This initial forming of the child had effects that were obvious for many years afterward. Perhaps even into adulthood. Is it worth a try?

Now let's go back and look over some of the "whys" behind Jarvis's recommendations. I will blend some of my explanations in with his. In my practice we have analyzed thousands of chemistries and have the benefit of equipment that wasn't invented in Jarvis's time. A lot of his suggestions were valid. He just didn't know the "why" behind all of them. I hope to contribute in this area.

Eliminate sugar. Everywhere you look you are beginning to hear that: Price, Page, Cheraskin, Yudkin, Newbold, Dudley et al. What does sugar do anyway? Jarvis breaks it down into relatively simple words, even if he does throw in some four-dollar words occasionally. Everything that is suggested in the line of diet or supplementation is directed toward influencing the endocrine system. The endocrine glands are primary stabilizers in keeping us in balance. These are glands like the pancreas (involved in controlling blood sugar), sex glands (involved in growth, development and reproduction), the thyroid (involved in energy production) and many more. They work like a team of horses pulling a wagon. There are two sets of reins, one for the left horses and one for the right. If one set gets ahead of the other, imbalance results, and there are two possible courses of action. Speed up the slow ones or slow down the fast ones. In the endocrine system we also have such a means of control. It's the *autonomic nervous system*. It is pulled by two sets of glands, the "left and right" of the horses, but in endocrine language they are called the *sympathetic division* and *parasympathetic division*. That's all the four-dollar words for a while.

You may have heard the phrase, "fight-or-flight reaction." This is what happens when the endocrine hormone adrenalin starts flowing. Adrenalin will flow in response to anger, pain, fear or any one of a number of other stimulating situations. The fight or flight reaction occurs when the sympathetic division of our endocrine system gets *ahead* of the parasympathetic (calming) division. This *same* reaction can get turned on by things like sugar and caffeine. In the case of sugar and caffeine, there is no tiger to fight or bully to run away from, but the body's "panic" buttons are all blinking. In a practical vein, this behavior is frequently seen at bedtime. "Calm down, calm down" parents are yelling as *their* adrenalin starts flowing. Then everyone becomes "sympathetic dominant" and spankings can result. Our nervous systems are of cave man quality, still geared for survival by the use of a club, and are interwoven with the endocrine system. When an artificial stimulant like sugar or the caffeine in coffee, tea or soft drinks turns on the sympathetic division, our "tempers" grow thin and we are ready for a prehistoric "attack." Actually, there is nothing but the cat asleep in the corner to attack—so *we* develop anxiety. It is hard (for adults and children) to cope with feelings that are *artificially* stimulated, so we tend to call it a "behavioral problem" and use drugs or spankings to counteract the situation. When sugar (commercial white or brown form—fruits not quite as much) goes into our body, the element chromium is released to keep the blood sugar from going sky high. If people eat excessive amounts of sugar (Americans average 110–120 pounds per person per year), more chromium is being used than is being replaced. The chart reproduced below of chromium content in the body, based on the work of Henry Schroeder, emphasizes how much chromium we lose during our first ten years of life—over 80 percent. If this chromium loss continues it can lead to a condition called diabetes. There are several ways to develop diabetes. This is only one.

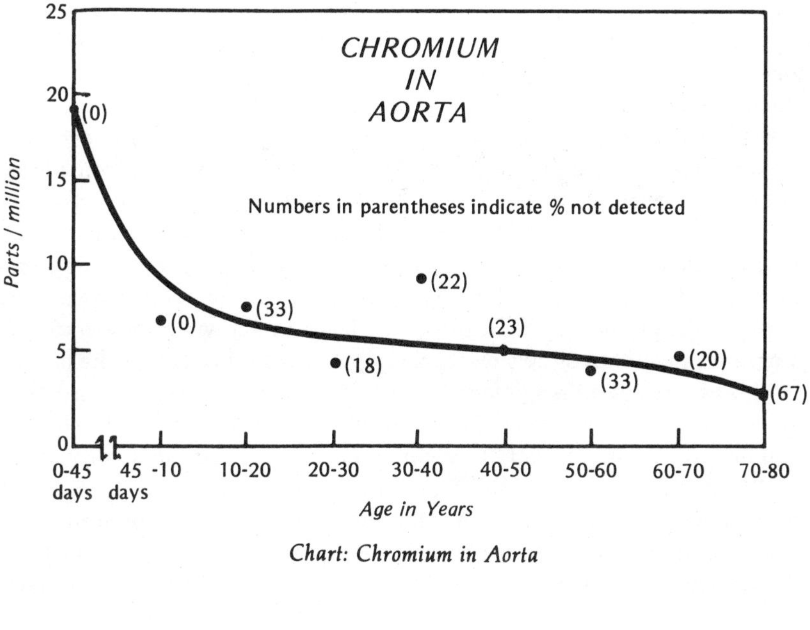

Chart: Chromium in Aorta

Jarvis saw sugar as interfering with proper grandular function, leading to inefficiency of cellular chemistry. Should the inefficiency continue it would lead to cellular breakdown, which we call disease. Not only do the endocrine glands of the body control the production of heat and energy, they also direct the constant rebuilding system we have within us. Every cell we have is in some stage of being born, functioning or dying. This is a never-ending process from birth to death, though we seldom pay much attention to it until we become sick.

A good example of this regeneration-degeneration cycle is the red blood cell. It is the primary oxygen carrier in the body. A red blood cell has an average lifespan of 120 days. At the end of the red blood cell's life, the spleen and liver break it apart (degeneration), recover the iron and a few other building blocks and then discard the worn-out parts into the intestines. Then reassembling (regeneration) begins. Iron, amino acids, and some new parts fuse, and behold, a new red blood cell is ready for another 120-day tour of duty.

If the two processes went on 50-50, we would probably live forever—but they don't. Here's the difference in people. If your regeneration replacement department were running 49 percent compared to 51 percent degeneration, you would be in great shape. If your replacement is only 30 percent and degeneration is going on at 70 percent, you will be said to be aging prematurely. There is no way to measure the percentages, but they are used to demonstrate a point. In my practice I use blood chemistry, trace element, vitamin and hormone analysis to get an *indication* of what this percentage might be. The *better* the chemistry, the better the efficiency of that degeneration-regeneration game.

We have developed some narrow ranges of values for these tests that seem to be associated with maximum efficiency. The mouth is considered to be the barometer of the body's health. Dr. Emanuel Cheraskin recently showed (in the Spring 1979 issue of *Annals of Dentistry,* an article called "Total Health: A Correlative Study in Stomatology and Electrocardiology") that there is a definite relationship between the health of the gums and the health of the heart as shown in the electrocardiogram (a test that shows electrical impulses running across the heart). In another article in *Angiology,* April 1968, titled "Effect of Carbohydrate Supplements Upon the Height of the T Wave in Lead I," he showed that he gave a "sugar load" to young men, then tested the quality of the health of the gums. An EKG was taken at the same time. Comparing before and after results he found that when eating sugar produced a bad change in gum health, there was a corresponding bad change in the EKG (indicative of the health of the heart). If sugar produced a minimum change in the health of the gums, then there was a minimum change in the health of the heart as seen in the EKG.

One of the indicators of gum health is to measure the amount of a fluid that is secreted in the gingival sulcus. The gingival sulcus is a crevice, or moat, around each tooth where the tooth and gum meet. The fluid that appears in this crevice is secreted by gum tissue around the tooth and *not* by the salivary glands. Dental experts pretty well agree that the amount of fluid secreted tells the health-disease story about gums. If there is zero secretion there is optimum gum health. The more fluid that's excreted, the worse the gum health. If heart health is also related to gum health, then perhaps a cross-section of total body health is seen by checking gums.

Using this gingival (gum) fluid flow as a guideline—the less the better—we have compared this flow to chemistry values. After watching patients' chemistries and comparing them to the gingival fluid flow, we have been able to find narrow blood ranges that are associated with healthy gums. It has been an exciting study, and the results are proving most gratifying.

From these tests, the EKG, fluid flow from the gums and blood tests, we are now able to tell what foods are good for people and which ones should be avoided. The surprising thing is that we all react a little differently when our chemistry is out of balance. We all require slightly different ways of achieving balance, but the notable thing is that the balance point (that is, the ideal level for the body chemistry) seems to be the same in almost everyone. There are deviations for children compared to adults, and there are subtle differences between men and women, but within these groups the balance point is amazingly consistent. I published an article on cholesterol demonstrating this point, and the *same story* seems to apply to all the chemistries we have studied.

Now, the point of all this: What upsets people's chemistry consistently more than anything else? Sugar. Which elements of the chemistry does it upset? I'll just mention the major ones in passing because you probably are not reading this book to get a comprehensive course in body chemistry. Major changes are seen in blood serum calcium, phosphorous, glucose, cholesterol and triglycerides when sugar is eaten. People can tolerate different amounts of sugar—both natural (fruits) or artificial (refined sucrose), and the blood tests can be used to find out how much sugar a person can eat and still retain the potential for good health.

One hundred and ten pounds per year is a lot of anything to suddenly drop from the diet, and this should be done with professional help if there is to be a smooth transition. The Academy of Preventive Medicine (10409

Town and Country Way, Houston, Texas 77024) has hundreds of members—MDs, DOs, veterinarians, dentists and chiropractors—who are aware of the value of proper nutrition. If you're interested in professional advice, this organization will furnish you with names of health professionals in your area. The reason I mention this is that if you are on a relatively high sugar diet and convert overnight—Bam! Withdrawal. Sometimes this withdrawal is uncomfortable enough to put you right back on sugar. "Oh, I felt terrible," "I had no energy," "I had a headache"—sound like heroin withdrawal? It's not quite as severe, but if you are not expecting it or don't have a "cushion diet" to help you through—oh, wow! *Cushion diet* is a term I just made up. There is no one cushion diet anymore than there is an *ideal diet* that fits everybody. I mean by *cushion* that substitutions of honey for sugar can be made, and types of proteins, fats, and carbohydrates that suit your chemistry best can be recommended. Nothing magical, just a helping hand through a transition to better eating habits.

Why eliminate wheat? Isn't it the staff of life? Actually, the biblical "daily bread" was made from millet, with flax and buckwheat as flavor enhancers. The wheat we eat today is relatively new to human consumption. It is a hybrid of ancient wheat. A lot of people do better "clinically" if they eat rye or corn bread in place of wheat. This is especially true of the pregnant woman, according to Jarvis. He says that the pregnant woman is more apt to get an imbalance of the autonomic nervous system if she eats wheat. Other grains won't do this as much.

Jarvis mentions the famous Wisconsin experiment of 1906 performed by S.M. Babcock. Babcock divided cows into three groups, feeding each group on the complete ripe plant of each test food. The three foods were oats, corn and wheat. Granted, cows have an entirely different digestive system than humans, but the results stimulated changing patient diets in a similar fashion. Those cows fed corn did well and produced normal calves. Those fed oats did moderately well. Those fed wheat developed rough coats, were irritable and produced premature, undersized calves. Most calves from the wheat group died within a few weeks, and those that lived were "fussy and hard to raise."

Jarvis next found that, given a selection of grains, birds would not eat wheat. He gave chickens a mixture of grains and found that the chickens either ate the wheat last or left it behind.

Transferring these ideas to his pregnant patients, he found that babies were more vigorous (*not* hyperkinetic) and appeared healthier by all standards when corn muffins, corn bread and rye bread were substituted for wheat in mother's diet. This was the test that *really* counted, and the indications are that people *and* animals may do better on grains other than wheat.

Why no milk? Boy, does this catch people off guard. For several decades milk has been one of the basics in our diet. Jarvis said that it formed a hard, undigestible curd in human stomachs, whereas it had the correct pH (acid level) for good digestion in a calf. He found that taking kids off milk frequently resulted in the disappearance of postnasal drip. This has been noted by many pediatricians recently. I know of several who take milk out of the diet of *all* their patients, but they want it kept hush-hush because of the big "where do you get your calcium if you don't drink milk" question. Where did we get calcium during the 10,000 years when we didn't drink cow's milk? From the foods we eat. Actually, in my body chemistry practice I see low calcium levels in about 6 patients in every 100, and I see *excess* calcium in over 60 percent.

What calcium are we talking about? There are two places that must be considered if we want to know the state of calcium in a patient. Blood chemistry furnishes one calcium guideline and the "elemental bioassay" (hair analysis) furnishes the other. Blood shows what is available to the cell, just as the corner grocery store has what is available to you. You must look into your kitchen to see what you have on your shelves, and in like fashion we need an indication of cellular stores. We look at an analysis of hair for an indication of cellular stores. Hair is *not* really dead tissue. Many people think it is dead because you don't say ouch when it's cut. There is an active two-way transport system in a hair strand, and it is the only protein extension of the body that has trace elements (manganese, copper, iron, etc.) attached to the protein in approximately the same concentration found in body tissues. Since each internal tissue varies in cellular composition, hair is a composite, or cross-section, of cellular activity. Blood is the same. Blood in the brain is not identical to that in the liver, but we accept blood from a vein in the arm as a standard for comparison. The blood test is also a composite.

When I first started testing trace elements (about 1968), I didn't know much about how to interpret the figures I got. No one else knew much either. Pooling knowledge has helped, but the greatest help has been watching individual patients change as we treat them. Our laboratory has now processed half a million individual trace element analyses, and we have learned much by observation. The scientific literature suggests avenues for investigation, as for instance: "Zinc is involved in insulin formation." Another comment from the literature might read, "Excess calcium blocks the activity of the zinc ion." In watching patients' chemistries we found some people had high glucose (blood sugar) with no dietary reason for it. Sometimes low zinc was present. Upon adding zinc we would see the glucose return to a better level. We learned something. What if the diet and the zinc were both good? Here's where we learned a lot about calcium and milk. If the blood sugar was high, zinc okay and calcium from the cellular aspect was high, then perhaps the high cellular calcium (determined by hair analysis) was blocking normal zinc activity.

But where did the calcium come from? In some cases it was from hard cheese, but in most cases it was from milk. Eliminating milk from the diet would lower the cellular calcium and eventually help an elevated glucose come down. Next, we found a really interesting phenomenon that was happening in the blood serum. Many times the blood calcium was *low*. How could it be low when the cellular analysis said there was an excess of calcium? It is simple when one looks at the body as a total mechanism designed to correct its own problems. When the cells became contaminated with too much calcium, the body knew it had to correct the situation. To do this it would lower the blood level of calcium.

This relative deficiency in the blood would cause the excess calcium to be pulled out of the cell so it could be excreted by the serum. Where does serum excrete extra calcium? One method is via the saliva. You may find it as tartar (or calculus), a stony barnaclelike substance that collects on the teeth. This is the stuff a dentist removes when he cleans your teeth.

So in these cases if I looked *just* at a blood test I would think the patient was calcium deficient and recommend calcium supplements. If the cellular (hair) test were high in calcium I would do my patient more harm than good. If both the cellular analysis and the blood were low in calcium, then *definitely* I would need to give calcium supplements to correct the problem. Jarvis didn't have all these analyses to worry about when he drew his conclusions, but guided by his suggestions, and following up with actual testing, I have found that his conclusions were valid.

Since milk was suggested to be the biggest source of inactive calcium, I began to ask, *why* is it inactive? Two reasons have been pointed out. Calcium is not transported as a mineral by itself. A chemical unit called an enzyme is needed for calcium to perform properly. The temperature of pasteurization kills this enzyme (catylase). Heat also converts the active form of calcium into an inactive form. These terms (*active* and *inactive*) are the only ones I know that accurately describe what we see happening in the chemistry. In the body the situation is similar to what mine was one day as I boarded a Continental Boeing 727. The stewardess saw my black case that I always carry, and since it looks just like the ones the pilots use to carry their dirty underwear, she said, "Hi—are you one of our Continental pilots deadheading?" (Deadheading is riding free.) She mistook me for a pilot. Pilots are usually tall, dark, handsome, suave and debonair, so I could see it was a natural mistake. I have sat in the driver's seat of a 727 and I can reach the brake, clutch and accelerator—but no way could I fly one of those babies.

This is just like the inactive calcium situation. Active calcium can sit in the driver's seat of an enzyme system (energy producing) but it can't operate it anymore than I can fly an airplane. Maybe magnesium or zinc could activate the enzyme, but as long as the calcium is sitting in the driver's seat, they won't be able to. If the pilot were standing beside me he couldn't fly the plane with me sitting in the seat either. This is the mechanism by which high levels of calcium seem to interfere with normal metabolism.

I picked up something else from my practice that led me to believe that Jarvis was right. We have our patients fill out a health questionnaire when they enter the practice as a new patient. For those who are going through the body chemistry program I started watching the number of symptoms they listed (each yes answer indicated a symptom) and comparing this to their chemistries. It didn't take long to find that high cellular calcium levels (determined by hair analysis) were associated with a higher number of yes answers on the questionnaire. A yes answer indicated a disease symptom was present or had been present at one time. In other words, the sicker patients had high cellular contaminations of calcium. This brought to mind an old saying I had heard. I have wondered if it may be more true than I had expected. Ever heard that "aging is calcification"?

There were other things about milk that made us question its use. In some 50 different publications a Bridgeport, Connecticut, cardiologist (heart specialist), Dr. Kurt Oster, wrote about milk as a primary factor to be considered in heart disease. The mechanism took several years to figure out, but he has established it and developed a technique for reversing the problems created by cow's milk.

Xanthine oxidase is an enzyme (small protein molecule) present in cow's milk that is absent from human milk. In raw milk it passes through our intestinal tract and is not absorbed. After homogenization the little protein sacks that hold xanthine oxidase are destroyed, and the enzyme can be absorbed from the intestinal tract and enter the blood stream. Here, over a period of years, it tends to injure the blood vessels—sort of etch them—causing a chemical change in that part of the vessel wall. This chemical change progressively causes the degeneration of the vessel wall (Oster lists the chemical steps) and allows calcium to deposit, aiding in hardening of the arteries. Oster found that folic acid and vitamin C given together would change that condition and give his patients improved heart and vessel health. Vitamin C was used at around a gram (1,000 milligrams) daily, and the folic acid was used at 60 to 80 milligrams daily. The recommended daily allowance for folic acid is less than one milligram. One milligram may keep body and soul together, but what about requirements for healing after a heart attack? Oster's results have been exceptional.

The American Society of Experimental Biology examined Oster's findings once, and in a long report quoting the literature, they said they could see no way for the xanthine oxidase to get from the intestinal tract to the blood stream. Oster then set up more experiments to identify the antibody to xanthine oxidase in the blood stream. An antibody is basically just what the word says. It is a body (or enzyme) that is "anti." Antibodies are warriors produced by the body, and each has as its sole purpose the destruction of one potentially damaging invader—in this case, xanthine oxidase. Oster reasoned that if a person had never been exposed to xanthine oxidase he would not have the antibody that works against it, and if he had, he would. He developed a test for the detection of the antibody, but where could he test it on people who had never been exposed to homogenized milk? He selected the Masai, a tribe of Africans characteristically close to seven feet tall and known to drink lots of fresh milk as well as the fresh blood of cattle.

In Masai country, homogenization of milk has *never* been practiced, so if Oster's theory were correct, there would be no antibody to xanthine oxidase in Masai blood. He went to Africa to test his theory and their blood. He was right. No antibody. *Everybody* he tested in the United States had the antibody.

Oster's discoveries over the past eight years have been impressive and informative. If the condition of the heart is related to the health of the gums as mentioned before, then how does the folic acid Oster uses affect the gums? In the 1976 *Journal of Periodontology* there is an article by Richard Vogel et al., showing that the gingival crevicular fluid flow that we discussed earlier is reduced when patients are given four milligrams of folic acid daily. Do you think we should consider a separate list of recommended daily allowances for people *not* in ideal health?

Stimulated by these findings I started testing blood for folic acid and its "partner," vitamin B-12. These two factors work as a team. In the past, I have found that taking pills without knowing where you are going gets things out of balance. People who take vitamin B-12 routinely—even in as *small* a dose as 14 micrograms daily (drug stores sell 1,000 microgram vitamin B-12 tablets *without* a prescription)—can make their B-12 levels excessive, while pushing their folic acid levels low. Folic acid and vitamin B-12 work like a teeter-totter. If folic is given without B-12 I have seen the folic acid go up and create a vitamin B-12 deficiency. I read in several textbooks that vitamin B-12 tablets were *not* absorbed by the body. To test this I checked the blood of my staff and patients. Funny thing, it's remarkable what you can see when you *look!* We found out that even the smaller dosages of vitamin B-12 create a disturbance.

Within two weeks of testing my staff and a few patients suspected of having vitamin B-12 and folic acid imbalances, strange things happened. I was using 10 to 20 milligrams of folic acid with some people (much smaller than Oster's dosages) and 20 micrograms of vitamin B-12 with others. On that small dosage of vitamin B-12 we saw tremendous drops in folic acid. But the folic acid didn't do much to the vitamin B-12 level. At 30 milligrams of folic acid we began to see a drop in vitamin B-12 levels. This concerned me. If Oster was using 60–80 milligrams of folic acid, what was happening to his patients' vitamin B-12 levels?

There was one way to find out. I called him. He said that he had not been testing vitamin B-12 levels routinely because they had not proved to be a problem during his initial studies. He said he would check several patients and call me back. Later he called to report what levels of vitamin B-12 his patients had, and they were *all* satisfactory.

What was happening? Did the high altitude of Colorado affect the vitamin B-12 levels? I doubted it.

Several months later the answer appeared. We tested a patient who had heard of Oster's work and was taking 30 milligrams of folic acid daily. I expected to find a low vitamin B-12 level—but didn't. Then it dawned on me. This patient—as *all* of Oster's patients—had had a heart attack. Not only that, but he was taking blood-thinning medication. Back to Roe's book, *Drug-Induced Nutritional Deficiencies.* Guess what? Blood thinners reduce the body's store of folic acid. Here was the answer. If a person is on blood thinners, his requirements for folic acid are dramatically increased. One other obscure comment I found added insult to injury. Not only does homogenized milk furnish the xanthine oxidase that can attack the blood vessels, milk also blocks the absorption of folic acid.

One thing that is a relatively common treatment for fatigue is a vitamin B-12 shot. Folic acid serves as a transport system for B-12. When a flood of B-12 comes in (as from a shot or pill) the folic acid transport system is used up quickly and we have elevated vitamin B-12 levels, folic acid is going down, and hemoglobin is going down. Why do you take B-

12 shots? To *raise* the hemoglobin (because vitamin B-12 is a component of hemoglobin manufacture).

What's happening? Hemoglobin formation requires several steps that are as much dependent on folic acid as on vitamin B-12. When the system is unbalanced by giving a dose of one part of the requirements without a measured knowledge of what the body really needs, severe imbalance can be created. What I'm saying is, don't go messing around with your own body if you don't know for sure what you need. One-a-day type vitamins are not apt to get you fouled up, but taking *megadosages without measurement* is what's dangerous.

I have one patient who thought he needed lots of vitamin B-6. I was testing his blood because I, too, thought he needed it, based on his symptoms. You should have 2–4 mg in the blood. He had over 90. This was way, way, way out of line. I had the serum retested, then asked the patient. He was taking half a dozen 50 mg tablets daily. He had overdosed. Vitamin B-6 at even 200 mg daily can have a diuretic effect and wash out an enormous amount of valuable trace elements.

B vitamins work together in a relatively narrow ratio. They have latitude and can accept a 100 or 200 percent deviation, but to elevate one thing from 3 mg to 90 mg is a 3,000 percent imbalance. He did it to himself—trying to help. I don't criticize people for trying to learn about maintaining their own health, but I try to stress moderation when it comes to taking a bunch of supplements. I may put a patient on 8 or 10 pills a day to start with, but I have 8 or 10 reasons—something measured in trace elements, blood chemistry, hormones, vitamins. There is an imbalance that is evident from an analysis as a basis for what I do. Megadoses have been used in the medical field for some years with great results, but leave the big bullets to the big guns. Leave it for those who have experience and evidence for what they are doing.

Any other comments on milk? Looking at our blood tests on patients we can see an obvious change in some areas, subtle changes elsewhere, but the main thing we see is different changes in different people. We all react a little bit differently. One unfortunate comment, though, is that all the changes that occur when we take people off milk are improvements.

Perhaps the most serious change milk brings about is in protein metabolism. One way of looking at protein metabolism is that it is a *combination* of the way the body breaks down meats, then turns around and builds up human body protein. This is an area that is superimportant in growing children. Childhood is the time that patterns are set up for life. If the blood chemistry values we monitor for protein digestion (uric acid, blood urea nitrogen, albumen, globulin) get out of balance in a *child,* I initiate treatment immediately. I don't care to sit around and wait for the diseases to occur. Imbalances in this area are associated with leukemia (cancer of the blood), collagen disease (cellular cement coming unglued), early heart problems (we know of a 15-year-old girl who had a heart attack last year) and a variety of other diseases that are not nice. I don't like to see the stage set for these things, especially when the treatment is relatively simple.

From the technical point of view, we look first to zinc, magnesium and their coworkers, then to supplementation to help the protein metabolism factors of the blood. A supplement of digestive enzymes usually corrects half of the imbalanced blood factors. Dietary changes work on the other half. If protein digestion is incomplete, it usually means that step number one needs help. Step number one is in the stomach. Stomach acids break down our foods. When we have a deficiency of these stomach acids, incomplete protein metabolism results. What dilutes acids? Any fluid. When the chemistry indicates protein metabolism problems, restrictions are placed on liquid intake during meals. Especially milk. Volume for volume, milk dilutes the digestive juices more than water. This doesn't imply *no* liquid with a meal, but some people consume three glasses per meal of milk, juice, pop, water, some liquid to wash down the food. If this habit is changed to one small glass of water per meal there will be a remarkable change in the blood chemistry. A doctor once told me that he had never seen this mentioned in the professional literature. My only answer is: "Then no one ever looked for it in the blood."

Who wants to cut down on fluids? Who *has* to cut down on fluids? The only people who really "have to" are those whose chemistries indicate incomplete protein metabolism. I suppose it would help *all* of us to increase efficiency, but that's a matter of choice. We show our patients where the problems are and what is involved in correcting them. There is a price to pay when the obvious is ignored, and most people find it easy to change habits when they know the reasons behind it. Drinking with a meal is a *social* development in our culture. It actually does very little to aid digestion, and in most cases works against it. This occasionally presents a problem (especially to those addicted to milk), but when they see their chemistry changes and feel other changes, it suddenly sheds a different light on the problem.

I'll point out a couple more things about milk and then we can move forward. In some areas there are reports of using estrogen- (female hormone) type substances in cattle to increase milk production. These areas also report that the estrogens are passed on to the consumer in the milk. Boys stop growing when their testosterone (male hormone) levels begin to build up. Estrogen from these injected cows had been implicated in retarding male hormone production. Boys in these areas were found to grow a little taller and be more effeminate. Local authorities recommended cutting down on milk consumption.

Other things are passed on to humans. Penicillin in animal feed has been passed on to humans through milk drinking. The problem here is that penicillin in small amounts can create allergies in some people. Some day you may need penicillin. Whatcha gonna do? If milk is *really* desired, a transition method that is satisfactory is to use cream and dilute it with water, three parts to one part, four parts to one part, or five parts to one part. This is okay. This can aid in absorption due to the fats and be helpful in this way. This is good in cooking too, at the four-to-one dilution. Baby bottles? Yes, diluted cream can be used here as a milk substitute. You might want to add a bit of honey. Later we will spend more time discussing honey.

Let's continue with Jarvis's check list. Next is to eat cheese. In monitoring blood and trace element tests we have noticed a lot of people don't do too well with *hard* cheese, but most people do well with *soft* cheese. What's the difference between hard and soft? I recommend the "finger test." This is a simple test *and* reasonably accurate. The equipment is inexpensive and readily available. Poke the cheese with your finger. If your finger bends first, it's a *hard* cheese. If your finger sinks into the cheese without bending, it's a *soft* cheese. You will find Monterey Jack, Colby, cheddar, and Longhorn to be hard cheeses, and Brie, Munster, Edam, and Camembert to be soft cheeses. In those people consuming too much cheese for their body, the cellular calcium level will be elevated. This is indicative of excess inactive calcium. Earlier we referred to this as calcium contamination. This can cause inefficiency due to its ability to replace magnesium, zinc and other minerals that are needed to activate energy-producing systems. People with that type of calcium contamination are the people who need to stop eating hard cheese. Once again, it *doesn't happen to everybody,* and the degree of the problem differs among individuals.

"Eat corn bread, corn muffins, cornmeal mush, fried cornmeal with butter and honey." There is a whole lost art in corn cooking that has given way to fast foods over the past few decades. Talk to grandmother and find out about these. My wife wrote the cookbook *Out of the Sugar Rut,* in which she includes corn recipes. She found many other references to corn cooking, so I know recipes are still around.

The recommendation to eat rye is another story. One hundred percent rye bread is hard to find, and if you do, you will learn it has a tendency to be crumbly. Here compromise may be the best you can get. Eighty percent rye should be acceptable. Actually, the term that should be emphasized here is *whole* grain. Many grains can be used separately or in combinations. Millet, flax and buckwheat are still around, but you don't hear much about them. Get daring; experiment.

Next, Jarvis says to eat one egg a day, minimum. The chicken egg is a good example of a "complete" food. It must be complete, it produces a whole chicken doesn't it? Any of the numerous ways to prepare eggs are acceptable, and remember that it isn't the egg that gives high cholesterol. It's the sugar, etc., as we discussed earlier.

Liver, heart and tripe are recommended, but we must use certain cautions that were not needed 30 years ago. Some cattle are raised in fields where pesticides and insecticides are found in the plants they eat. Many of these substances are stored in the liver. The liver acts as a filter that removes harmful things from the bloodstream. It might be worthwhile to look around for a meat source from cattle raised on pesticide-free pastures. It wouldn't hurt if they were free from injections of growth hormones. These factors are becoming important to a number of people to the point that some commercial enterprises are offering better quality beef. Calf liver should be better in these respects than old-cow liver. Some people don't care for the taste of liver, but do like liverwurst. This is an acceptable compromise, according to Jarvis.

Two raw vegetables daily shouldn't pose much of a problem, and "nuts to you" might be a good slogan during pregnancy. What's a nut? Probably the first thing we think of is the peanut. Peanuts are *not* nuts. Nuts grow *above* the ground, and peanuts grow *below*. Peanuts are classified as legumes, or beans. They are high in carbohydrates and can contribute to unnecessary weight gain. Nuts (cashews, almonds, pecans, sunflower seeds) are getting to be awfully expensive now, so why not look into bulk purchases? They keep well, and you can save a great deal of money buying 25 pounds at a time, compared to the two-ounce package.

Jarvis says avoid citrus fruits. But you can eat grapes and apples or drink cranberry juice. Don't we need vitamin C? We usually think of citrus fruit and vitamin C in the same breath. Yes, vitamin C *is* important, and we recommend that most of our patients take additional vitamin C. The dosage is based on blood and urine tests for vitamin C. Citrus fruits contain citric acid—an acid *not* digested well by humans. Jarvis found that the autonomic nervous system (our endocrine team of horses) is unbalanced by citrus. In blood tests on our patients, we see undesirable high blood serum calcium produced. This contributes to calculus formation on the teeth. If the calcium precipitates out of the serum in other areas—say into the joint structure of the arthritic—it is undesirable. In fact, anywhere excess calcium is deposited, it causes problems.

Let's talk about one of "mother's" problems for a minute. Morning sickness. This is as uncomfortable today as it was in the thirties. Jarvis recommended drinking a mixture of apple cider vinegar and honey upon rising. The formula has a few critical points. One is that you should use apple cider vinegar that is made from the *whole* apple, not just pressed from the cores. There are probably several companies that make it, but Heinz is the only one I know of for sure. Put two tablespoons of apple cider vinegar in a four-ounce glass, add honey until it becomes palatable, then fill the glass with water. Sip this prior to rising or shortly afterward, and sip it during meals. One glass should last all day. For midday, try cranberry, apple or grape juice.

In our practice we have noted that pregnant women who have morning sickness are usually quite low in manganese. Frequently, we will give them manganese to balance their chemistry and have an improvement in morning sickness as a nice side-effect.

Another problem mother runs into during pregnancy is constipation. Jarvis found honey to be a great stabilizer without giving diarrhea. His starting dose was two teaspoons with each meal, taken by spoon as if it were a medicine. If that wasn't enough he would increase the dosage by one-half teaspoon. Another nice side effect of honey is that it has a soothing effect on the nervous system and can offer more restful sleep. He also found a carry-over into the autonomic nervous system of the baby by observing that the babies were seldom fussy. He felt that the whole autonomic nervous system is in better balance when mother ate honey as he prescribed while she carried the child.

Looking over menus of the world there appears to be a great variety of table delights available. Geography plays a big role in nutrition because food availability is directly related to weather conditions and crop potential. People from the mountains eat differently from people of the plains or the poles, yet there is one food that we have with us today that is held in esteem by all mankind. Honey. Since the dawn of recorded history honey has been mentioned by every race. It was always a crowd pleaser and still is.

Jarvis said of it once, "Honey is the world's most complete food." He, of course, was looking at it through the eyes of a medical man interested in prevention through building internal resistance. He saw many attributes in its contents and found many areas in which he could use it as a medicinal agent. He also noted a great deal of difference between the sugar in honey as compared to the sugars produced from cane, beets and corn.

Natural sugars are "burned" in the cells to produce energy. Most of these sugars contain a number of enzymes, trace elements and nutrients to help rebuild cellular structures. This is *not* true of sugars made from cane, beets and corn. As refined sugars became more popular and cheaper, from 1900 through the 1950s, Jarvis began to note new conditions arising in his patients. He looked back into former diets to see if he could find the answers. Honey seemed to be a *big* part of the answer. He looked at the whole diet profile and compared this to total patient health, but in order to learn about a subject it is often best to remove it from the landscape and examine it under the microscope. That's what we're going to do with honey for a few minutes. We're going to look at it in relation to many disorders that resulted when certain deficiencies were produced.

Natural sugars like the ones found in honey burn slowly and continually within a properly supplied cell. Dextrose in honey is absorbed rapidly and does not need to undergo a chemical process called inversion before it can be put to use in the body. Another honey sugar, levulose, is a *real* slow reactor. Together they produce good absorption for rapid revitalization of a tired body without producing the big *upswing* of blood sugar that leads to endocrine turmoil.

Refined sugars, on the other hand, react violently by comparison.

Refined sugar burns like straw within a cell compared to natural sugars burning like coal. This flare-up provides quick (though brief) stimulation without bringing any nutrient value with it. (I define *nutrient* as that which the body can use to rebuild its worn-out tissues.) This sudden stimulation jars the system and puts undue stress on the liver, kidneys, lungs, vascular system and nervous system, which Jarvis says leads to high blood pressure, diabetes, arthritis and many other disorders termed "degenerative diseases." The human body is constantly tearing down old tissue and replacing it with new. When the tear-down process is faster than the buildup, we dissolve into a condition known as degenerative disease.

We have already mentioned that all of our red blood cells are replaced every 120 days. This is a degeneration-regeneration process carried out by the liver and spleen. Some tissues turn over even faster. Dr. Ralph Steinman of Loma Linda University has told me that a chemical (condroitan sulfate) within the dentin (second layer of the tooth) has a rebuilding rate of 50 percent every 60 minutes. That's *really* rapid regeneration. All this requires raw materials (or nutrients) as well as energy. With refined sugars we have energy but no nutrient.

What does honey supply? Mother Nature differs from man in that man singles things out. Man looks at life as a rifle looks at a target. For a bull's eye. Mother Nature works like a shotgun. That is why you find two sugars, dextrose and levulose, in honey. These supply energy rapidly without causing an excessive elevation of blood sugar. These sugars create energy that can be used to form new tissues in the body. Honey also contains raw materials (amino acids and minerals) needed in the formation of enzymes. It has biological ferments that are active in energy release. The mineral content is shotgunned for a variety of uses. Copper, iron and manganese are helpful in oxidation within the cell as well as being necessary for hemoglobin formation. Hemoglobin carries the oxygen from the lungs to the tissues so that energy can be released. Other elements include silica, chlorine, calcium, potassium, sodium, phosphorous, sulfur, aluminum and magnesium.

Vitamins are abundant in honey. It contains B-1, B-2, C, pantothenic acid, pyridoxine and nicotinic acid. It contains more of these than most fruits and vegetables, and has another advantage to boot. Whereas spinach loses 50 percent of its vitamin C in one day after it is picked, honey maintains its full strength of vitamin C and the other nutrients indefinitely. "A perfect food from the medical point of view," said Jarvis, "it should be taken with each meal to insure continued good health . . . and . . . will help greatly in maintaining the health of your body and the balance of your nervous system."

Professor H.A. Schuette of the Department of Chemistry at the University of Wisconsin felt much the same way that Jarvis felt. He was one of the early advocates of the necessity of trace elements for optimum metabolism. "I would like to call your attention," he wrote in 1950, "to the presence of these newer essentials, copper, iron, and manganese, of which there seems to be a larger quantity in dark honeys than in light ones."

Schuette went on to say, "The pollen of many flowers has a higher vitamin C content than almost any fruit or vegetable. One of the most important facts established is the somewhat surprising one that honey is an excellent medium for vitamins. This is not true of vegetables and fruits that lost a large percentage of their vitamin content within 24 hours after being picked."

Honey has advantages for us in cooking. It has a germicidal effect because it is a "magnet" for water. Germs need a certain amount of water within their cells, and honey tends to draw water out of the germs, resulting in their death. Its magnetic attraction for water also tends to make breads and baked goods stay moist and edible longer. Since this property exists (primarily due to the levulose), honey should *never* be stored in a refrigerator or cool place. It needs to be in a warm, dry place in a tightly closed container. Honey can destroy bacteria by the same method described above. It pulls out the water, but in addition, its acid nature is not conducive to bacterial growth.

Applying this water attraction property to humans, honey can be a big help with bedwetting problems. By the time a child is two years old it is time to develop bladder control. A few months later night bladder control usually follows, but there are cases that go on for years with nocturnal accidents. Jarvis found that by limiting fluids after 5 P.M. and by giving the child a teaspoon of honey at bedtime, bladder control can be improved.

What's the mechanism behind this? Jarvis had noted that nervousness was nearly always present in bedwetters of three years of age and older. He usually found nail-biting, temper tantrums, thumb-sucking or infantile speech present. These are all symptoms related to an imbalance in the autonomic nervous system that we discuss periodically. The upset autonomic nervous system is that team of horses in which one horse gets ahead of the other. In bedwetting, temper tantrums, etc., one would expect to see an overactive sympathetic division. The counterpart—the parasympathetic division—must be encouraged and the sympathetic slowed down before any of these symptoms can reverse. The application of honey here is excellent because it tends to be a sedative to the overactive sympathetic nervous system. This technique also encompasses honey's ability to attract and concentrate water. Together, these reactions bring about improvement in many bedwetting cases. After control has been established, the bedtime honey can be used as needed. Experience showed Jarvis that children's parties and heavy play activity just prior to bedtime predisposed children to bedwetting, so these are times when honey should be used.

Honey can play an essential role in growth and development when used daily during the first years of life. Mother's breast milk is best for the child with rare exception, but there are times when artificial milk must be used. According to Dr. Ralph Steinman of Loma Linda University, the best artificial milks are those made from lactose. Corn syrup—like Karo— is usually recommended as a sweetener, but Steinman, Jarvis and many other notable authorities suggest that *honey* be used in its place. There was a group of doctors at the University of Minnesota and at Chicago University who studied the differences between corn syrup and honey in artificial milk. They were watching for changes in the blood sugar levels, calcium absorption, effects of vitamin D with both, magnesium absorption and a host of other clinical observations.

Quoting the work of Drs. Schultz and Knott of Chicago University, "Very interesting results were obtained with honey." Children were given samples of various sugars and their blood sugar levels tested at 12, 30, 60, 90, and 120 minutes after dosing. "During the first 15 minutes honey was absorbed most quickly of all the sugars except glucose. Even at that, honey did *not flood* the blood stream with an overabundance of sugar. It maintained both a steady increase and slow decrease in blood sugar until the initial level was reestablished. This response to honey is presumably levulose. Honey is quickly taken into the blood because of its dextrose content, while the levulose, being somewhat more slowly absorbed, is able to maintain blood sugar. Honey has the advantage over other dextrose-containing sugars since honey does not cause the blood sugar to rise to higher levels than can be easily cared for by the body."

From my work in body chemistry I can sympathize with these men's concern for a stable blood-sugar level. Blood-sugar levels are elevated in almost all cases of rampant decay as well as advanced cases of gum disease. I have yet to see a case of either brought under control until the blood-sugar level was improved. In looking at the laboratory reports going from my laboratory to my physician colleagues, I can see that they too have the same problem. Not only is diabetes associated with high blood-sugar levels but patients suffering from arthritis, bursitis, cancer, heart disease, high blood pressure, cataracts, etc., etc., carry high blood sugar levels.

Henry Schroeder, MD, has recently pointed out the importance of the element chromium in the control of blood sugar. His studies point out that we lose more than 80 percent of our stored chromium during the first ten years of life. Many important elements like sodium, potassium and magnesium can be reclaimed by the kidneys, filtered out and returned to circulation. Chromium cannot. When the blood sugar goes up, chromium is released into the bloodstream to help bring the blood sugar down to the proper level. Then the chromium is excreted in the urine. When we put refined sugars into our bodies, the blood sugar goes up higher than it does with natural sugars, resulting in a greater loss of chromium. The best way to reduce chromium loss is to put foods into the body that do not cause drastic elevations in blood sugar.

Returning to Schultz's and Knott's work, they concluded that honey was easily digested, well tolerated by infants and aided constipation without causing diarrhea. This was one of Jarvis's major points too. As you remember, he found that in cases of constipation, two teaspoons of honey at bedtime usually corrected the problem. He varied the dosage up or down one-half teaspoon as needed.

Schultz and Knott knew of the importance of minerals in addition to vitamins, proteins, carbohydrates and fats, and stated, "It is not enough to supply these minerals in food, it is important that the largest part of them be retained by the body for its own use." In order to find out whether honey or corn syrup served better in assisting mineral absorption, they and two other doctors ran 120 test periods with 14 infants. They measured the amount of calcium and magnesium in the food, then the amount of calcium and magnesium in the urine and feces. The difference showed how much was retained by the child. Several types of milk were tested, as well as varying amounts of vitamin D. The primary factor that altered mineral retention turned out to be whether honey or corn syrup (Karo) was used. All tests indicated that calcium retention by the child was higher when honey was the sweetener than when corn syrup was used, regardless of the other variables. Magnesium is of relatively low concentration in bone but is highly responsible for bone density. Magnesium content is high in soft tissues and helps to prevent muscle and nerve irritability.

Results showed that honey with powdered skim milk provided 16 milligrams per day magnesium retention, while corn syrup and milk yeilded only 0.4 milligrams per day with the same kids. Honey provided a 40-fold (4,000 percent) increase in magnesium retention over corn syrup.

As a side-effect of their experiments, this team also noted that diaper rash occurred when corn syrup was used, and it quickly disappeared when corn syrup was replaced by honey. Infants fed honey rarely showed the formation of gas in the intestinal tract. This is because the rapid absorption of honey prevents fermentation from taking place. Fermentation is what produces gas.

In studying the many advantages of honey in the artificial milk it appeared to Schultz and Knott that one to two teaspoons in an eight-ounce feeding mixture produced the best results. Should an infant become constipated, they increased the amount of honey by one-half teaspoon. Likewise, if looseness of the bowels was noted, the amount of honey was decreased by one-half teaspoon.

You may remember that Dr. Archie Kalokerinos spoke of the use of vitamin C during teething. Dr. Jarvis adds to this information a bit about the autonomic nervous system again. As with most problems, teething is associated with an overstimulated sympathetic division of the autonomic nervous system. To relieve the symptoms of teething in a child less than one year old, Jarvis prescribed one-quarter teaspoon of honey at bedtime. Give the child a few sips of water to wash away any residual honey left in the mouth. As the child gets older, the amount of honey is increased until one teaspoon is reached. This is as high a dosage as should be needed. Effects are usually visible within less than an hour. Jarvis found that the pain associated with teething was parallel to the tissue phosphorous level. Honey diminishes the tissue phosphorous level, and the pain usually subsides.

Jarvis had a long list of honey's medicinal properties. Some of these have already been discussed, but I will repeat them just to have them all together in a group. Probably one of the most practical uses for a parent toward the end of the day is the calming effect honey has on kids *and* adults. Some children become fretful after the evening meal and become more so as bedtime approaches. A teaspoon of honey with the evening meal will produce a calming effect within an hour, thereby soothing the nerves of both parent and child.

Schultz and Knott had mentioned the disappearance of diaper rash when honey rather than corn syrup was used in baby's formula. Jarvis agrees and adds to this the use of honey in controlling bowel problems. The remarkable thing about honey is that it can correct constipation without giving diarrhea.

Some children have weak digestive systems and frequent stomachaches. Since honey is so soothing to the stomach it tends to lessen the stomach-ache problem. This is probably due to the digestive enzymes, biological ferments and rapid absorption.

An excellent cough medicine can be prepared from honey. There are many narcotic cough medicines available today, but those of you who would like to save stronger medications until they are really needed can try this formula. Boil one lemon slowly for 10 minutes. This will allow you to get more juice out of it upon cutting it open. It also softens the rind. Squeeze the juice into an eight-ounce jar and add two tablespoons of glycerine. Glycerine can be purchased at most drugstores at a very nominal cost. Drugstore jargon for two tablespoons is one ounce. Stir this, then add six ounces (12 tablespoons) of honey and stir again. Tighten the lid and store this in the medicine cabinet or kitchen, but *do not* put it in the refrigerator. Always stir the solution before using it. The dosage is one teaspoon as needed. This could be every 30 minutes or every hour until it becomes effective, then once every three to six hours as it appears to be needed. This is very effective, safe for kids and does not upset the stomach.

Teething, as mentioned before, is a good time to think about honey. When teething creates the cranky kid, the sympathetic division of our old friend the autonomic nervous system is overdoing again. Pupils dilate, tissue phosphorous level goes up and inflammation appears, while peace and quiet exit. If the child is less than one year old, use one-fourth teaspoon of honey followed by a sip of water. As the child gets older, the amount of honey can be increased to one teaspoon. It takes about two and a half hours to see changes in the blood produced by the honey, but you should note a calming effect in the child in less than an hour. Sometimes this effect will last up to 24 hours.

Kids need to absorb the calcium they are eating for proper growth of bones, teeth, fingernails and hair. First, the calcium must be in the proper chemical form for absorption. Tests indicate that when foods are heated to high temperatures there is less absorption of biologically active ingredients.

The heat of cooking seems to produce some compounds of calcium that are not active for life-promoting actions, but they hang around and take up space. This I call "calcium contamination." More will be mentioned about calcium contamination in the chapter on hyperkinetic kids. The tests by Schultz and Knott indicate that far more calcium is retained when honey is used than when corn syrup is used. Remember that the magnesium—one of the really important elements in growth and development—was also better absorbed when honey was used.

There has been a deluge of articles about botulism and infant death during the past year (1981). Since Jarvis and Price had found so many attributes for honey, I thought it best to look into the situation. I found things like "botulism *could* grow in the intestines of infants" and " the spores can apparently develop." In other words, the authors are being cautious.

This looked like a simple enough thing to study, so we undertook some experiments. Honey in the comb was extracted with sterile instruments and incubated on several growth media. What happened? Nothing. Honey in the comb is sterile. As we checked raw, processed and filtered, and pasteurized honey, we found progressively more bacteria. Man is the contaminant. To go a step further, we inoculated raw honey with Clostridium and incubated the honey. The bugs died. There was no sign of gas formation. Gas is the by-product of digestion of Clostridium. These tests were not repeated a hundred times to form an absolute, but they are indicative that Jarvis and Price may be right.

I did find one interesting point. Much honey is mixed with "HFC," which is high fructose corn syrup. Our pathologist brought it to my attention that he had been asked to devise a test to distinguish "HFC" from honey to identify those unscrupulous people who are diluting honey with corn syrup and selling it as honey. There is no easy, reliable test to distinguish the difference. Maybe honey is not the real problem after all. It could still be man.

Another interesting tidbit was handed to me from La Leche League files. (If you are pregnant or thinking about becoming that way, contact them. They are one of the most valuable assets our next generation has.) The Food Research Institute of the University of Wisconsin at Madison published data on the botulism problem. They found that *all* raw agricultural products grown in soil—that is, fruits and vegetables—contain botulism spores. All.

It's hard to get away from botulism spores, but it is easy to see why I recommend buying honey from the keepers. Know your bees. Buy direct. No one wants to give their kids diseases, but I would suggest that this one has been blown a bit out of proportion. If we followed the University of Wisconsin's findings and tried to avoid all foods grown in soil, we would find ourselves with a bit of a food supply problem.

Jarvis once said, "For me, the crowning glory of honey is its medicinal value." He was talking about adults as well as kids when he said that, so I think we should scoop all these tidbits together and look at them in an orderly fashion.

First, the medicinal use of honey in babyhood. Diaper rash is noticeable within the first few days of life if corn syrup is used as a sweetener in formula feeding. Switching from corn syrup to honey (two teaspoons per eight-ounce feeding) will tend to eliminate most diaper rash. While helping diaper rash you will also be helping your child absorb more of the important minerals he needs. Calcium and magnesium were discussed in detail earlier in this chapter, but all the minerals (trace minerals included) will be absorbed better with corn syrup removed. This will be reflected in better growth and development. Another simultaneous side-effect is the control of constipation. Honey provides a gentle laxative effect without producing diarrhea. The "dosage" of two teaspoons of honey per eight-ounce feeding can be varied one-half teaspoon up or down according to whether more or less effect is needed. When honey is used daily in the feeding, it will help keep the autonomic nervous system in balance. The result of this is a happy baby as compared to a fretful one. When more effect is required, like when a child is whimpering at bedtime, one-fourth to one-half teaspoon of honey will produce a calming effect within less than an hour. This may be in conjunction with teeth—a fretful situation when the sympathetic division of the autonomic nervous system is in command. Half a teaspoon of honey may calm the upset nervous system for as long as 24 hours. When a cough appears, one of the best cough medicines is the one described earlier in this chapter. It produces the desired effect without the use of drugs.

As a baby transforms into a child some of the same problems exist, some new ones appear, and some are gone forever (like diapers). Well, they should be. Occasionally, bedwetting will be a problem even past five years. Jarvis found the use of honey in concentrating the urine to be an effective method of helping many bedwetting problems. Two teaspoons can be given at bedtime for a twofold objective. He found that occasional bedwetting was related to the excitement state of the child 30 minutes before bedtime. If the child had been around "company" and had played hard or become more than usually keyed up, an accident was more apt to happen. Honey calms the nervous system at the same time that it is demonstrating its magnet-for-water ability. Of course, it can be used for the "hyper" condition by itself without the presence of bedwetting. Sometimes that hyper condition is related to playing at an unfamiliar task that produces muscle fatigue in muscles that are not accustomed to the stress put upon them. This leaves the muscles tired and sore due to lack of enough blood sugar in the tissues. Honey produces an influx of sugar to these parts without pushing the total blood sugar level excessively high. The result nourishes the spent muscles and restores a sense of well-being.

Allergies are not the sole property of the child, but this seems like a good time to discuss them. Allergies have three basic elements, two that are subject to control—one that is not. Heredity, body chemistry changes, and autonomic nervous system disturbances are the big three. Obviously, heredity is the one that we can't change. There is ample evidence to suggest that allergic parents tend to produce allergic children.

What about factor two, the biochemistry? Where did this idea come from? In the 1940s there was an MD, Major Seymour C. Schwartz, assigned to the Medical Corps at William Beaumont General Hospital in El Paso, Texas. His men were troubled by allergies to the point that the problem got his special attention. After some discussion he found that many people living in that area had the same affliction but had found a remedy for it. Jarvis quoted Schwartz's findings and added that Vermonters near him had used the same treatment for years. What it amounted to was chewing the "caps" from the honeycombs *made in the vicinity.*

Caps are the ends of the storage tubes collectively known as the comb. When one side of the comb is cut off to let the honey out, what is cut off is the cap. Analysis of this portion of the comb shows that it is rich in pantothenic acid and many other nutrients. The bee gets its raw materials from pine and spruce bark primarily, but will use other bark if these are not available. Schwartz reported that the symptoms of hay fever would usually subside within three to four hours when the afflicted would chew one-half teaspoon of the caps for ten minutes, then either swallow the wax or spit it out. It's a little more effective if swallowed, but this is not essential. The chewing routine was practiced every 30 minutes until symptoms disappeared. Dr. Schwartz also emphasized the advantage of a complete lack of undesirable side-effects. Hay fever medicines usually produced drowsiness, which led to a whole new series of problems. No drowsiness is produced when chewing honeycomb. If caps are not readily available, a child can chew up a one-inch square of honeycomb to get a similar effect.

That sounded to me like *real* folklore. I couldn't understand why if it was *that* good all the allergists in the country weren't using it. My wife and I got some honey cappings "just to try." I admit I didn't have much confidence in the idea. A friend of Joanie's dropped by shortly after we got the cappings and asked what they were for. As fate would have it, she had never been able to sleep the night through during the summer months due to hay fever. We gave her some cappings to chew, and her nose began to dry up. Within a few hours she was cleared up and spent her first restful summer night in years.

This turned us on to the possibilities, so we started talking about it. Within a week my five pounds of cappings were gone, the bees were through making honey for the year, and 25 people were angry with us for running out. The next year we got 50 pounds of cappings and started using it on body chemistry patients. I have seen no side-effects from its use in two years, and have seen many allergy problems either minimized or completely cleared up. Now I have people ask me: "Since this stuff is so good, why doesn't everybody prescribe it?" Well, now that *you* know, why don't you prescribe it?

Jarvis talked of an easy home test for allergy susceptibility. Squibb Company puts out nitrazine paper. This is a thin strip of test paper that changes color depending on whether it is in an acid or an alkaline solution. This test does give a good indication of the balance between your body's resistance and the stress that is being applied to it. Nitrazine paper is used to check the urine pH, a measurement of acidity or alkalinity. Pure water has a pH of 7.0. A reading below 7.0 is acid, and higher than 7.0 is alkaline. When the body's chemistry is at *maximum resistance* to allergies, the urine will test *acid* on the nitrazine paper. Matching the color of the test paper to the color chart on the box will show a yellowish color equal to a reading of 5.0, more or less. When the paper is turned blue by urine, it is alkaline—a pH of 7.5 or above. This blue color (meaning alkalinity) indicates that the body is *susceptible* to allergy attack.

Now, what things make the urine turn alkaline? Foods that will turn the urine alkaline (indicating susceptibility) are white bread, cakes, crackers, donuts, wheat cereals, citrus fruits and milk. In other words, sugar and wheat products which are found in most processed foods will make the body more vulnerable to attack from allergies. Exchange corn and rye products for the wheat, honey for sugar; avoid citrus and milk, and you can start rebuilding resistance.

Foods aren't the only things that tear down resistance. Physical and mental factors play a measurable role. Prolonged physical work, prolonged mental work, emotional upsets, unproductive worry, an unhappy environment, exposure to cold and some drugs or medicines will produce an alkaline urine. Jarvis suggests one treatment that can help correct the situation, while the slower process of changing foods is taking place. The use of apple cider vinegar—one to two teaspoons with each meal—will help change the chemistry and let you produce a yellow nitrazine test again. Straight apple cider vinegar is quite a belt, so you may want to use one of Jarvis's other ways to get apple cider vinegar down. You can put two teaspoons of apple cider vinegar in a glass, add honey until it is palatable, then add four ounces of water and stir. Sip this with each meal until the urine test turns the nitrazine paper yellowish. Cranberry juice or cranapple juice will alter the pH favorably, but not as effectively.

Chapter Ten

Why Raise Holey Teeth?

Dental decay was rare in most primitive tribes. Why are we plagued with it? Lifestyle. One that can be changed to produce unholey teeth. All we have to know is where decay actually comes from, and we can figure out how to control it. If the ancients could do it, so can we.

The health problem that affects more children today than any other is dental decay. Estimates, advertising and actuality don't always meld. It is estimated that 95 percent of our children today have active dental decay. It is estimated that fluoride has reduced much of the decay in our society. Dr. Fred Jones recently did a follow-up examination on the original fluoride study done 20 years ago in Tulsa, Oklahoma. Twenty years after the study there is *no* significant difference between the original "two groups." Pedodontists (specialists in dentistry for children) tell me there is still rampant decay in many three-year-olds. I have heard speakers say that decay is a disease of childhood. From my practice I would say this is true only when compared to my denture patients. Regardless, dental decay is a problem in children, and dental decay is *ugly*.

Sometimes we tend to laugh at dental decay, much as we do at ourselves when we get a parking ticket. We got caught. We all fudge once in a while on feeding ourselves and not feeding parking meters. Once in a while you expect to get caught, but then what does it cost us? For a buck or two we are forgiven for our parking sins, and for 15 or 20 bucks we get absolution for eating something we shouldn't have. The tooth is filled and all is forgiven.

Or is it? This might be the case if decay were the *only* effect of what we did, as with the fine for a parking meter violation. Unfortunately, violation of enamel is not due to the food that stuck to it. If that were true, then brushing and flossing would eliminate tooth decay. There are 120,000 dentists in the U.S., and most of them spend most of their time filling teeth. I've heard it stated that if every dentist in the U.S. worked 24 hours a day for a year on nothing but decay, there would still be cavities left unfilled. Brushing and flossing help, it's true, but evidently that's not the crux of the problem.

Dental decay attacks by two routes. Internal and external. There are myriad members on both teams, so sometimes I wonder how we can possibly get through life without being plagued by decay. Then I remember the observations Dr. Weston Price made. There were areas that he studied where he found only *one cavity per 1,000 teeth* in skulls. That means that at the end of life's journey the teeth were still in nearly mint condition. Did people living hundreds of years ago have an advanced civilization? Did someone from Atlantis rise from the sea and give them magic toothpaste? I doubt it. Theirs was a completely different way of living. A way of living that is impossible to duplicate today, and who would want to? Houses without heat or air conditioning, having to spend all day trying to catch game or gather grain for the evening meal—does this sound preferable to today's way of living? No, not to the majority of people. But there is a way out. There are things that we can do to increase our resistance to dental decay without having to move out on civilization.

What we have to do is identify dental decay and find out where it comes from. I mentioned external and internal factors. We can look at these factors as two groups, but there is an overlapping that fuses them into one concept. In the final analysis, the best thing we can do is blend all the parts into a way of life that we can live without having to think about it minute by minute.

External factors that influence dental decay include bacteria, food in the mouth, how the teeth fit next to each other, exercise and stress. Internal factors that resist decay might include heredity, hardness of the tooth, the foods we eat, hormones, vitamins, minerals, metabolic shields and the fluid transport through the teeth. All these things make it sound as if there is more to dental decay than brushing, don't they? Yes, the tooth has to be considered as an organ, like the liver or kidney, before we can totally understand how to cope with the problem of decay. The three basic divisions of the tooth (enamel, dentin and pulp chamber) all mutually depend on each other, and fluids from one part pass to the other parts.

These concepts of external and internal factors are far different from what I was taught in school. I feel that dentistry owes a great debt of gratitude to Dr. Ralph Steinman of Loma Linda Dental College in California. He is a researcher who *looks*. His thoughts are not confined to the "what's always been accepted" philosophy that governs so many researchers. Dr. Steinman destroyed my sand castles of picturesque logical concepts with one tidal wave of knowledge in 1973.

I was taught that food decomposed around the teeth after a few hours and produced acids that dissolved the enamel. After the initial break in the enamel, bacteria could march down into the dentin, breaking enamel rods and proteins into little bitty pieces, leaving in its wake the soft brown "gunk" we call decay. Only by removing the decay and replacing it with silver-mercury, gold or plastic fillings could the process be stopped. The speed at which cavities developed might differ in different people, but there was no way to halt the progress of decay. We could help prevent it, however, by giving children fluoride to make their enamel harder.

Let's look back again—remember Dr. Weston Price of several chapters ago? He found all those decay-free skulls and taught us the importance of diet in the control of decay. He found one isolated island where decay was virtually unknow until an epidemic hit. During his travels he had an opportunity to visit this island two times over a 15-year period. On the first visit the islanders were free from decay. On a subsequent visit he found some teeth rotted half away, but the brownish-black areas of "decay" were solid—not the soft mush dentists usually find. It was as if an epidemic of decay had hit the people, then went away, allowing the half-decayed teeth to heal. Checking on the island's history it was found that traders had come to the island to obtain copra. They offered the people white sugar and white flour in exchange and kept an active business going for several years. Soon the need for copra vanished and so did the traders. During the time of abundance of sugar and white flour, decay flourished on the island. When the people were forced to resume their native diet the decay process reversed. It is reported that Price noted this in the 1930s.

In about 1958, Steinman began presenting his revolutionary concepts and the research to back it up. We spoke of the acid attack on the enamel due to the decomposition of foods. He looked. He measured the amount of acid produced on the teeth of rats fed a good diet (no sugar) versus that produced on a poor diet (62 percent sugar). Much to my amazement he found *more* acid produced on a *good* diet than with the high-sugar diet. There went sand castle number one.

The "acid attack" could not produce dental decay. In his office I saw microscopic pictures of enamel from both test groups and found surprise number two. Where there was sugar and a relatively *lower* acid content, there was a *great deal* of *etching* on the enamel surfaces. Where there was a *high* amount of acid, there was *no* etching visible on the enamel.

"How can this be?" I asked Dr. Steinman.

"Decay is a systemic disease," he replied. "You are trying to find the cause in 'local factors.' Dental decay comes from within, not from without. Certainly, local factors play a role, but they are not the *initiating* factors in dental decay."

"If acid is not an initiator," I asked, "what about bacteria? Obviously the *high sugar diet* was related to decay and enamel etching, though I don't understand why, but what about bacteria?"

He showed me some of his research and some of Dr. Kite's, in which both researchers implicated bacteria in decay. Both researchers raised animals in *germ-free* environments and *neither* produced decay *regardless* of the diet. Microscopic sections of the teeth of these animals showed chemical changes that set the stage for decay, but decay as such was not present.

"Okay," I asked, "so you can show this on a rat's tooth, but what does that have to do with human decay?"

Dr. Steinman explained that "every biochemical process of decay identified in man is found to be identical in the rat." He personally had studied over twenty biological processes and found rat decay and human decay to be identical. In fact, the *only* difference between the two is the *speed* of the reaction. All life processes go on faster in the rat than in man.

As in a game of chess, I moved one more pawn forward. "What about heredity?"

"I'm sure heredity plays some role in decay susceptibility, but it can't be proven. In fact, the opposite has been proven. In a study of 256 children versus their parents we found a *negative* correlation between parent and child where decay-proneness was measured. Current diet played an overpowering role here and superseded hereditary predispositions. Foods can reverse the activities of the endocrine system, you know."

Yes, I knew that, and saw his point. In my next attempt to bridge the gap between our two states of knowledge, I led with a trump. "Doesn't fluoride make the teeth harder and more resistant to decay?"

"You are partially right. Fluoride makes teeth harder, but [here he got out more research reports] the *hardness* of enamel has *no* relationship to resistance to decay."

The foundations of another sand castle crumbled, and I could visualize the walls disappearing underneath another tide of knowledge. I played my last card. "Fluoride does decrease decay, doesn't it?"

"Yes, but I'll have to explain the action of the parotid gland and the fluid movement through the tooth before you can see how fluoride works."

Fluid movement—through a solid tooth? This guy has lost his mind. After eruption, the tooth is a solid body that just *sits* there in the mouth. Oh, those old sand castles.

Dr. Steinman spent the better part of an hour explaining how fluid moves from the pulp chamber *through* the dentin, *through* the enamel into the mouth. This fluid is similar to fluids found between the cells in the rest of the body. He explained that he had injected acriflavin hydrochloride—a radioactive material—into the abdominal cavities of rats, and was able to recover it in the "solid" structure of the tooth within minutes.

This is what happens in a healthy individual. This explains why acid sitting on the tooth did no damage. Acid has to get *into* a tooth to do damage, and with a fluid flow running from the pulp chamber through the dentin in six minutes and on to the surface of the tooth in less than an hour, acids, etc., from the mouth can't swim upstream, so to speak. Steinman went on to explain that, by altering the function of endocrine glands, that fluid flow could be reversed such that the tooth sucked bacteria, acids and other things *from the mouth into the tooth.* He had many slides that demonstrated fluid movement in both directions.

"Can you alter the direction of flow?" I asked, for this seemed to be the ultimate goal if dental decay were to be controlled.

"Yes, we can," he began, "simply by changing the diet. We have found a lot of foods that cause the fluid to flow inward, and many foods that stimulate it to flow outward [which is optimum]. Most of the 'flow-in' [decay-producing] foods are the refined foods, as you might suspect. Sugar, refined flour and convenience foods are the biggest part of those contributing to creating a condition favoring dental decay. Generally speaking, proteins, fruits, vegetables, grains and nuts favor the tooth's defense against decay. There is a fine line about heredity here too. About age two or three years, the permanent teeth are forming within the jawbone. If there is a deficiency of vitamin C, D or A during calcification, a tooth less resistant to decay will be produced. This is not really heredity, but the next best thing to it."

"Are you ready to fit fluoride into the picture yet?" I asked.

"Almost," he replied. "You need to have one more biology lesson first. Haven't you wondered what the mechanism is for altering fluid movement through the tooth?"

"Yes."

"Well, that involves the production of a hormone that Dr. John Leonora and I have isolated. We call it *parotid hormone* because it is produced by the parotid gland. We usually think of the parotid as a salivary gland producing saliva, but it also produces a hormone. Now, what stimulates the parotid gland to produce its hormones? Like most endocrine glands, its production schedule is controlled by a master gland. The hypothalamus releases a hormone which in turn stimulates the parotid to release its parotid hormone. When the parotid hormone is at its proper level, the fluids travel from the pulp chamber through the dentin, through the enamel, and into the mouth. Refined sugar has the ability to *stop* the hypothalamus from functioning properly. Less hypothalamus activity means less parotid activity, and that leads to reversal of the fluid-flow in the tooth. Now—here come fluoride. Fluoride stimulates the action of the hypothalamus."

"So dental decay *is* systemic—not topical—and so is the action of fluoride?"

"Right."

"Have you done any other tests to show that dental decay is systemic?"

"Yes. In fact, here are a few reprints of our work." More papers, more data, more information that pushed me farther and farther into the biochemical approach to dental problems.

* * *

I had seen an ad in a dental journal telling dentists that soft drinks go through the mouth so fast that they could not possibly cause dental decay. In my practice I was not able to confirm this freedom from decay. Soft drink drinkers seemed to have cavities in proportion to how many drinks they drank. Steinman used stomach tubes to put sugar solutions similar to soft drinks into rats' stomachs. This involves placing a small tube down the throat directly into the stomach. This is a sort of mouth bypass. Guess what? The test animals got decay at the same rate as "control" animals who ate the same amount of sugar by mouth. Maybe the tube leaked. In other experiments sugar solutions were *injected* into the abdominal cavity—close to but *not* in the stomach. Guess again? Yes, the same number of cavities. Now injection is *certainly* "going through" the mouth too fast, yet here was the decay. This experiment is the one that *totally* convinced me of the systemic nature of dental decay.

Other hormones play a role in decay susceptibility. Perhaps hormones explain why there is so much decay in teenagers. The estrogen-testosterone levels are high one day, low the next and normal the next. As these hormone levels change, many other body chemicals, like potassium, sodium, phosphorous and calcium, change. These alterations tend to make teeth more susceptible to decay. Thyroid levels affect both dental decay and gum disease, but the really bad part is that an imbalance either way—high or low—can cause an upset in the chemistry that will increase disease susceptibility. If we look closely, we can find our old friends, the sympathetic and parasympathetic nervous systems, again. In an article on hormone effects, Steinman points out that decay is more predominant when the system is "sympathetic-dominant." He used synthetic drugs to make the sympathetic system dominant, then other drugs —parasympathetic stimulators—to counter the effect, and found that there was far less decay when there was good balance between the two. It's the same story told in sprinklings throughout this book: Balance the endocrine system. Here it is applied to dental decay.

Minerals have their day too. In some studies quoted by Steinman—actually performed by Anderson—copper, iron and manganese were added to a decay-producing diet, and the decay rate was almost abolished. (Copper, iron and manganese are active in intracellular oxidation, the energy-producing reactions that prevent bacteria from charging down the dentin tubules.) Steinman's work also measured the magnesium losses in the tooth as the tooth became more decay-susceptible. Indeed, the magnesium level dropped to nearly zero as the experiment continued.

With all this talk about trace elements and fluid flows I began to wonder, so I asked, "When does decay start and where?" (To myself I thought: Prepare thyself for destruction, oh sainted sand castle.)

"Teeth decay from the inside out, you know—don't you?" The look on my face was one of oh, not again. "If you want to plot the course of dental decay you should look at the slides we made. Rats were put on a decay-producing diet, then each day a few were sacrificed and slide sections made of their teeth. The first step in dental decay is the same as with disease in any part of the body. There is a change in *function.* In this case it means the fluid flow is altered from flowing from the inside out to the outside in. Next we see inflammation occurring in the pulp chamber next to the dentin. Watching the enamel and dentin under a microscope we can soon identify the loss of magnesium, copper, iron, manganese, ATP, ADP, sulf-hydro groups, acetycholine, etc., etc.—a whole bunch of complex chemical life-preservers disappearing. All this activity goes on within the pulp chamber, spreading to the dentin and finally to the enamel—*prior* to the time you spot a tiny cavity on your X-ray film."

Oh, that's a heavy. "You mentioned 'external factors.' Just what were you studying?"

"Stress and exercise."

In one of Steinman's experiments the same diet was used on animals where one group was confined and the other group could run in its cages as much as it desired. The diet was one that encouraged cavities to develop. On identical (poor) diets, the exercise animals developed 4.8 cavities per animal compared to the nonexercise rats, who developed 14.9 cavities per animal. Does exercise effect health? It certainly made a big difference in the decay rate. Confining an animal produces stress, and it is hard to distinguish the lack of exercise from the stress produced. There are many ways to produce stress—heat, cold, noise, lack of sleep—but almost any condition that could scientifically be called stress will produce similar systemic changes. Corticotropin (a cortisone produced in the body) is elevated and there is a change in sodium and potassium distribution. There is also an alteration in the amount of sex hormones. This can produce a big change in the chemistry of the body. My conclusion from this conversation was that there is much intertwining of external and internal factors.

* * *

As complex as dental decay is scientifically, it boils down to simplicity when we look at cause and cure. The ancients and the people today who have not been touched by foods of commerce are not bothered with dental decay. What's at fault? We are. Our lifestyle. We are reaping what we sow.

Can we get out of this mess and still live where we do? Yes. A few simple rules of nature can put us in good dental health. You can buy good foods at most large grocery stores now. You can find whole grains and learn to cook with them. You can have cakes and cookies that taste good without having to resort to sugar. Overcooking is a big problem and not hard to overcome. Later, my wife Joanie has a chapter that covers how to accomplish these changes successfully.

Dr. Price came to us as a "missionary from the primitives" to tell us how we can stop our epidemic. He says we can reverse physical degeneration by adhering to age-old principles. The principles exclude most fast foods and move you up to the world of gourmet flavors. As our teeth become healthier, so will the rest of our bodies. We are the captains of our souls. We are the masters of our fate.

Chapter Eleven

Why Raise Jumping Jacks?

The hyperkinetic kid never lights. He is off the walls and ceiling, and uses the floor only as a place to clean mud off his shoes. Everyone will agree that the hyperkinetic kid is an Ugly Kid. There are several ways to create a hyperkinetic kid. Once you know what they are, you can begin to reverse the process.

Probably one of the toughest jobs a parent can have is to keep track of a hyperkinetic kid. It takes all but radar to keep up with him. No pattern exists, he just goes, goes, and goes—and usually gets into trouble on the way. One solution I've heard is: "*You* take the kid's vitamins and give *him* your tranquilizers." But I don't think any of us *really* thinks that drugs get to the cause of the problem, and few of us like the idea of having drug-dependent children.

There are many ways to develop a hyperkinetic child, but it has been an interesting observation to me that they all look alike from the chemistry standpoint. This is contrary to almost any other affliction that registers changes in the chemistry. For the most part it is a person's individual response to an upset chemistry that leads to a disease profile. In other words, chemical values by themselves are *not* diagnostic. A blood sugar of 120 mg % does not guarantee that a person will develop diabetes or gum disease, one, the other, both or neither, yet at some time both the patient with gum disease and the diabetic will probably have this blood-sugar level. Many people have that level and develop an entirely different disease, but the upset in glucose (blood sugar) metabolism is just a supporting actor—not the main character.

For some reason unknown to me, nearly all children labeled *hyperkinetic* have a *magnesium* level of between 8 and 12 parts per million, as seen in the hair analysis. What gets me is that the range for magnesium goes from around 3 parts per million to more than 800 parts per million. Why such a *narrow* range for the *hyperkinetic* kid? The fact that there is a magnesium deficiency makes good sense because of its involvement in nerve-impulse transmission. There are several elements that are needed for proper management of nerve impulses. Calcium, magnesium, manganese, sodium, potassium and lithium are some of the essential ingredients. When magnesium is either low or its activity is bound up by another element, improper impulses result. With a *low* magnesium level, the nerve-impulse-firing mechanism is superirritable. It acts in "hair trigger" fashion, firing too rapidly and at times firing when it should not fire at all.

Daily we are bombarded with thousands of stimulations from our environment. If we were acutely aware of every background sound that entered our ears we would soon go nuts, or at least become hyperkinetic. Listen now. Is music playing? How many instruments? Are people talking somewhere near? Radio, stereo, television, cars driving by, wind blowing, house squeaking, air conditioner or furnace running, the dishwasher, or just a pounding in your head because you are trying to block out all of the above? (Magnesium helps filter these impulses so we respond to those that are meaningful.) The hyperkinetic child's nerves *are* reacting to all of the above. Sounds are not the only thing that the hyperkinetic kid is responding to. He is also responding to things he has eaten and to radiation that may bombard him most of his waking hours. Can this condition be corrected? Yes—*if* you want it to be corrected.

That sounds like a threat, doesn't it? Well, actually it is a *challenge*, because our everyday mode of living is responsible for a lot of the hyperkinetic activity seen. Here again, a part of your lifestyle may have to be changed. Is it worth it? This is for you to decide.

Examine the causes presented here, compare them with your lifestyle, and most important of all, figure out *who* is in control of your household. Hyperkinetic children tend to dominate the scene wherever they are. Often it is easier on you (parent, teacher, babysitter, etc.) to let them have their way than to expend all *your* energy just keeping them in line for a few seconds. Remember, though, that once the chemistry is improved many of those problems can vanish so quickly that you wonder if someone changed kids with you when you weren't looking. This is not promising miracles or selling a gimmick. It is merely an attempt to put things in order. Hyperkinetic behavior is *not* normal. It's ugly.

Kids can be fun. Try this and see if it doesn't make a big difference in personal warmth both to and from your hyper kid. It should come as no surprise now to hear the terms sympathetic and parasympathetic divisions of the autonomic nervous system. These have been cropping up in about every other chapter. Well, it works here too. One factor we face is the overactive sympathetic nervous system. What have we seen in past chapters as the chief cause of imbalances? Sugar. Sugar primarily means refined white, brown, turbinado and yellow-brown but not necessarily the natural sugars. Natural sugars like those in fruits do *not* get an automatic clean bill of health, because they too are sugars and require the same elements for proper digestion as refined sugar. If the child is low in magnesium, chromium and zinc, he may have trouble metabolizing natural sugars. For the more severe cases, a doctor can provide analyses and interpretation of data, but the first really big step is to *look to the obvious.* They are: ice cream, candy, pop (one of the biggest sources because it includes so many drinks), pastries and the junk foods that provide calories but a minimum of nutrients. So often I hear young mothers say, "But he won't eat anything else." The child in tow is usually preschool. My favorite dig is: "Does *he* go to the store and buy it?"

"Of course not. He's only three years old."

Well—who's in charge? Records reveal that only a minimal number of children voluntarily starve to death when faced with the dilemma of choosing between good food and starvation. Another weather-worn woe is: "But he *likes* it."

My comeback for this one is: "Are you going to buy his marijuana for him because he likes it?"

The light dawns: Who's in charge?

How do you get kids off sugar? By substitution, *not* cold turkey. Cold turkey produces antagonism, but substitution combined with explanations and love can have remarkable results. Honey can be substituted in cooking, but *be ready* before you dive into an elimination program. This is *so* important. Get a good cookbook on cooking with honey and whole grains. Buy the ingredients, experiment on yourself and when you are ready, gently slip into something more cookable. *Cooking With Love and Wheat Germ* by Jean Kinderlehrer (Rodale Press), is a good recipe source, and of course, I feel my wife's book *Out of the Sugar Rut* is the best. For kids ten years and over, give them half to three-quarters of a teaspoon of unprocessed honey at bedtime. Under age ten, use one-quarter to one-half teaspoon. Ages and dosages here are *guidelines*—you may want to adjust one way or another for personal reasons. Just remember: if a little bit is good, a lot may have the *opposite* effect.

Let's take a look at some isolated cases, but *not* at the expense of losing sight of the overall picture. A seven-year-old dental patient of mine exploded onto the scene after an absence of about a year. Nice enough kid, not noisy, not hostile, just mobile. If I would take three-fourths of a second to reach for an instrument he would flip over on his stomach (not a comfortable position in a dental chair) and knock all the instruments from the tray onto the floor, then in an assisting manner flip out of the chair, knocking the light in circles while helping pick up the instruments. While on the floor he might as well check out the air and water hoses, for after all, they crawled out of an interesting looking cabinet that probably had other toys nestled within. You know, three or four seconds of this can make an old man out of you, let alone alter blood pressure, schedules and feelings of brotherly love.

An idea that I learned early in the game of dentistry with children is that if I touch a child timidly he is going to take control of the whole office instantly. If I pick him up in the reception room—especially upside down—he figures this is going to be an adventure and that I'm not scared of kids. What physical contact could I use to get this kid's attention? A club? Oh, no, there are laws. I scooped him up off the floor and planted him back in the chair saying "Thanks, buddy, for helping pick up the instruments,"then promptly swung my leg across his chest. "Oh boy, this is fun," you could see beaming from his eyes.

"Now let's look at a tooth or two."

"Where did you get—?" This presents a fine opportunity to slip a mouth mirror to the molar area. I like the word *get;* with kids it forms just the right shape at the corners of the mouth to allow a mouth mirror to slip practically unnoticed clear back to the molars. When the teeth find something between them, the surprised mouth opens for an instant—long enough for me to slip the mirror 90 degrees with my fingers so that I now have a prop accepted by the teeth and not licked by the tongue.

I've been in dentistry enough years that it doesn't take me long to spot a cavity, much less 16 of them. My first glance revealed about 10 of the 16 and I came unglued. Knowing that having this many cavities at age seven is not the child's responsibility, but that of his parents, I gathered up my holding leg, composure and sternest look, then stomped off into the reception room. "Mother" knows me as a gentle, quiet, kindly, compassionate sort of fellow who likes to fill teeth. Now it was my turn to explode onto the scene. Sitting alone in the reception room Mother looked up and smiled as I entered. She looked like the television ad mother waiting for the dentist to say "Johnnie only has 16 cavities" so she could twinkle her eyes and retort, "It must be the Crest."

"Do you know what you've done to this kid?!" I demanded without breaking stride. Her smile oozed back on her face as if she were an astronaut being pulled against the force of gravity. "This kid has cavities—gobs of cavities. And he's only *seven* years old. I have seen skulls that have been buried in mud for centuries that have better looking teeth. You've rotted out the most resistant structure God put in the human head—and not in seven years, but in five, because most of these teeth didn't erupt until he was two years old. I say *you* because I know who does the grocery shopping at your place—and it isn't the kid. If the mouth is the barometer of the body's health, baby, you've got a typhoon on your hands, because *rotten* teeth mean *rotten body*. And *you* did it."

Baffled, bumfuzzeled and beaten, Mother began to sputter, "It's the grandparents. They give him candy."

Nice to have grandparents—nice bunch, aren't we? Broad shoulders, lots of pictures and, inevitably, candy. Then I sat down.

"Candy is part of the problem, yes, and I'm sure that between the two of us we can change the grandparents' attitude toward that. In fact, if you don't tell them today, I'm going to." (I know them.)

"No, no," she sputtered. "You've got to be gentle with my mother. She *means* well."

"Candy alone can't do all the damage that has been done to that boy's body. Want to talk about it?"

"Why, yes. What can I do?"

I wasn't sure whether her intentions were to improve the boy's health or to dampen my wrath. No matter, we proceeded. I did something I rarely do. I had a 10-minute consultation about dietary changes without an analysis. Usually this approach is *doomed* to failure. I feel the success we have had in balancing body chemistry is due to the fact that we *educate* our patients as to what blood- and trace-element chemistry means to them and how they can change it with dietary control. I decided to take a chance. Basically, I found that the child ate mostly canned foods at meals and high-sugar-content foods in between. Sugar has been suggested as one of the hyperkinetic causes, so Mother and I decided to change from canned foods to fresh foods and eliminate sugar where possible.

Three weeks later the boy came in for the first session of his overhaul. I was ready—storm windows up, instruments *far* from the chair, and my right leg limber for the "holding program." What a shock! He hopped into the chair, opened his mouth, and hardly moved a muscle during the next 60 minutes—60 minutes in which I repaired four badly broken-down teeth. He was a pleasure to have in the office—bright, inquisitive, but always ready to cooperate when it was time to work on the teeth. No muss, no fuss, no jumping around and—oh, yes, I forgot the amazing part: all this restoration and *no* anesthetic necessary. He didn't feel a thing.

Caffeine is another culprit in the hyperkinetic complex. Give the kid a cup of coffee? Not on your life! It will stunt his growth. Give him a cola drink. We have tested nearly 50 drinks for caffeine content and find that coffee is the highest. Commercial coffee, that you find in some restaurants, can run as high as 150 milligrams of caffeine to the cup. Soft drinks run around 40 to 50 milligrams if they are cola types. Lemon-lime types contain no caffeine, only sugar or sugar substitutes. Chocolate candy contains caffeine (actually thiobromine, which is a caffeinelike chemical) in addition to sugar.

How much caffeine does it take to create a response? This varies with the individual, but in some people 10 to 20 milligrams can cause detectable changes.

A few years ago we had a patient who had a mouth full of canker sores. She had some as big as a quarter under her tongue and had rarely been free of them for eight years. When we balanced her chemistry, the cankers dropped in size to just a few millimeters in diameter. She was comfortable and ecstatic about the change, but just as a personal challenge she wanted to see if she could succeed 100 percent. After an hour of carefully examining everything she ate, my only suggestion was that it might be that she was reacting to the caffeine in the glass of weak iced tea she had daily for lunch. Considering that one cup of tea contains around 50 to 60 milligrams of caffeine, I figured that she was getting roughly 8 milligrams in her tea. She stopped the tea, and within three days the cankers were *completely* gone. She remained free from them (except for brief times of "dietary sinning") for 18 months. At that time she moved and we lost track of her.

What are you going to drink? This is the biggest problem we face in balancing body chemistry because drinking is a *social* requirement, not a biological need. We may not need as much fluid intake as we have been led to believe. Take the instance of Dr. Vernon Nord. To test the fluid-need-theory, he drank only 40 cc of water (about one ounce) per day for a year. He explained that by far the largest part of our foods is actually water. Squeeze all the fluid out of a fruit, vegetable or meat, and what do you have left? Not much. The human body is over 90 percent water, so maybe there is enough fluid around. Hot weather and heavy exercise do increase our needs, but what I am referring to is the eight glasses of water frequently recommended even for sedentary people, to "flush" the body. What happened to Dr. Nord? He went through Dr. Ken Cooper's aerobics testing program in Dallas and came out in the top 2 percent of men under 30. Not bad for a 52-year-old grandfather!

It would be nice if the academic community would get interested in reports like this and test them scientifically. I am one man paying for my own research and cannot possibly accomplish the mountains of research suggested in this book.

Back to the drink. Sit down for breakfast in a restaurant—you know, yawning, bleary-eyed, adjusting to an upright position, and here comes a waitress. She's been up since 4 A.M. "Coffee?" she asks, and within the 0.36 seconds required for the fastest human reaction, you have a cup of coffee. Fast gals, these waitresses. Try dinner.

"For your main course?"

"Prime rib."

"Prepared?"

"Rare."

"Salad dressing?"

"Blue Cheese."

"Butter or sour cream on the potato?"

"Both."

"And to drink?"

"Nothing."

"No, I don't mean a cocktail. I mean a beverage with your meal."

"Nothing, thank you. I'll have water."

"Not even tea?"

"No, thank you."

"Well, we *do* have milk."

You get the feeling that if you don't give in and *drink* something she is going to yell at you—something like: "Look, dumb-dumb. If you don't drink coffee, tea or milk like everyone else, I'm gonna call a cop."

The one that I really like is the prepared waitress. She comes charging toward your table with a pot of coffee tipping your direction 10 paces away. "Coffee?" she threatens as she skids to a stop. Aware of the impending attack you put your hand over the cup. Scald! Or, if you have turned the cup upside down (to give time for an instant of conversation—like, no, thanks) she may stop, give you a "wrong religion" type of look and walk away without taking your order. That always makes me want to call out, "Does that mean I can't have breakfast?"

Go to a neighbor's and what's the most frequently asked question? "What can I get you to drink?" Well, that leads back to the original question. Do you *really* want to correct the hyperkinetic? We raise our kids to "Drink your milk, drink your juice, no, you can't have coffee, have some pop"—then all of a sudden, about face. Whaaat? This creates confusion in an already confused hyperkinetic mind. The only way over this hyperkinetic hurdle is to teach—to explain—with love. Love doesn't always increase acceptance, but it keeps you from beating the kid and saying, "Look, youngun. I'm going to do something good for you, even if it kills us both."

What's a good compromise? Water (for all its attributes) doesn't rank very high on the scale of social entertainment. Fruit juices (made from the whole fruit) mixed with carbonated water provide a socially acceptable beverage with a minimal amount of biochemical disturbance. Carbonated water is available at most grocery stores, is practically nothing but carbonated water, and is good for the Kool-Aid substitution.

Another idea for quenching your family's thirst is herb teas. Celestial Seasonings of Boulder, Colorado, makes some very good ones, and they are available in supermarkets throughout the country. Be sure to read the label, however, because a few of their teas contain caffeine. The herb teas are delicious alone, mixed together, cold or hot. Try different kinds of these teas until you find one all your family will enjoy.

Postum is delicious served both as a hot drink or iced, and it contains no caffeine or sugar. Fruit drinks can be made in the blender, using the whole fruit (add some water and a tiny bit of raw honey). Switch from regular coffee to the decaffeinated kinds, which are satisfying served either hot or iced. If you must have a sweetener, use only a little raw honey, no chemical-laden sugar substitutes, as these may be harmful to the body.

Despite all the advertising on how we never outgrow our need for cow's milk, I have seen a number of people whose chemistry improves when they avoid milk. Hyperkinetic kids are among them. They develop an addictionlike thirst for milk and have great difficulty giving it up. Apparently, milk blocks the absorption of magnesium and many other trace elements. This is another reason for the low magnesium levels in the hyperkinetic. Here again, milk is not the sole cause of hyperkinetic problems, but kids can improve rapidly when it is avoided. Where will they get their calcium? The same place they've always gotten it. Refer back to chapter nine for the milk discussion.

There have been a good many articles in the newspapers about the work of Dr. Benjamin Feingold. His feeling is that the additives and coloring agents in foods contribute to hyperkinetic behavior. According to Jacqueline Verrett of the Food and Drug Administration, we consume an average of 1,200 additives and food-coloring agents during 24 hours of "ordinary American diet." Dr. Feingold has had success in controlling hyperkinetic behavior by eliminating foods that contain these agents. A recent article testing Feingold's theory pointed out that these foods produced hyperkinetic behavior even with the additives *missing*. With reports becoming available—such as Verrett's material—I see no way in which we can say additives and coloring agents are helpful or safe where health is concerned. The additives may or may not be the real culprit, but nonetheless, if the foods that Feingold recommends eliminating (mainly junk foods) *are* avoided, improvement in hyperkinetic behavior should be noted.

Another inexpensive, effective method of treating the hyperkinetic kid is to limit his exposure to *inside* radiation and increase his exposure to *outside* radiation. Dr. John Ott of Sarasota, Florida, deserves a lot of credit for discovering another cause of hyperkinesis. He has pointed out the new disease called *malillumination*. What that means is underexposure to sunlight. His research of over 30 years has shown him that plants, animals and man all require radiation from the *sun* for proper health. He points out the importance of "nocturnal radiation," or radiation that is emitted during the night from the Van Allen Belts, which are out in space around the earth. The sun's effects on the Van Allen Belts do not become apparent on earth until several hours later, thus the nocturnal influence.

Ultraviolet radiation has long been thought to be harmful to humans, and we have been warned to avoid it. Dr. Ott's work shows that ultraviolet radiation is *necessary* for proper functioning of our endocrine glands. His latest book, and by far his best, is *Health and Light*. In his book he describes his struggle for acceptance of his theories and observations. He also describes many useful changes we can make in our lifestyle to gain better health. He has found a relationship between light and cholesterol, calcium deposits, dental decay, cancer, and even the *hyperkinetic child.* Dr. Ott has produced a movie (he is an authority on time-lapse photography) demonstrating the effects of pink fluorescent lighting on children's behavior. Schoolrooms lighted with pink fluorescent lighting produced extremely hyperactive children. He next changed the lighting to full spectrum lights, and within a few weeks, he photographed children with *normal* behavior patterns. These were the *same kids.* Full spectum lighting is available in most cities of 100,000 or more and can be special ordered in almost any city.

The best-balanced light exposure, though, is outdoors. But there is a problem here too. If the child wears eyeglasses made of *glass,* the eyes will not get the necessary ultraviolet stimulation. Glass filters out the ultraviolet light. Plastic lenses will allow over 90 percent of the ultraviolet to get through to the eyes. The retina of the eye is the primary center of activity. Ultraviolet exposure to the retina in the eye produces a balancing effect on the endocrine glands. There are now a variety of plastic lenses available, but the one designed by Dr. Ott is made so that a total distribution of the sun's rays can penetrate equally. This is available in regular lenses or in contact lenses. After reading the results of Dr. Ott's experiments with light, one is convinced that outdoor activities are quite healthful. They are necessary if you are going to gain control over the hyperactive complex.

Now that we can get a bit of outdoor exposure, what can we do about inside radiation? Dr. Ott deserves another credit for his discovery that radiation from the television set is another contributing factor to the development of the hyperkinetic child. He started out with animal experiments based on an idea presented by two pediatricians at the American Academy of Pediatrics in New York City. Their report was covered in the November 6, 1964, issue of *Time.*

The pediatricians were noting funny symptoms in kids whose blood tests proved negative for infections and suspected diseases. Some kids were nervous, some tired, some fatigued, others overactive, but *all* the kids cycled through *most* of the symptoms at one time or another. They told 30 sets of parents to cut out television for the kids. Twelve enforced the rule, and the symptoms were gone in two to three weeks. Eighteen of the families cut television to about two hours daily and saw results after five to six weeks. Eleven families dropped the restrictions and the kids got the same old symptoms again.

Dr. Ott put laboratory rats in front of a television set for what is considered average time for kids, 6 hours daily during the week and 10 hours daily on the weekends. Two cages were placed in front of the television, one shielded from the screen with a lead plate, the other shielded with black paper. Neither set of animals could see the visible light. Only nonvisible radiation could penetrate. The sound was shut off. From Ott's book: "The rats protected only with the black paper became increasingly hyperactive and aggressive within from 3 to 10 days and then became progressively lethargic. Even with the lead shield as protection, the other set of rats showed a small degree of abnormal behavior. Is there, in effect, radiation coming out of the television set?"

According to an August 1965 letter to Dr. Ott from the Electronic Industries Association, the National Committee on Radiation Protection and the International Commission on Radiation Protection have set a limit of 0.5 milliroentgen (mr) per hour at 5 centimeters from the television screen as a maximum acceptable safe level. A major television manufacturer was quoted in the press as saying, "The matter of the possibility of any harmful radiation from television sets was under complete control by the entire industry and sets were constantly being tested and double checked for any possible X-rays by the Underwriters Laboratories."

Dr. Ott goes on to tell that "when a representative of Underwriters Laboratories was questioned by the press on this point, he said that they had tested for electrical shock, etc., but he flatly denied that Underwriters Laboratories had tested for possible X-rays emitted from the sets."

From the political standpoint, Dr. Robert Elder, Director of HEW's Bureau of Radiological Health, testified at a congressional hearing that "small doses of radiation are cumulative and may cause genetic damage affecting future generations." In May 1967 General Electric recalled 154,000 television sets because of excessive radiation. Excessive—yes, if 0.5 mr is maximum, it was well to recall those. Some were delivering *40,000 mr per hour.*

The U.S. Public Health Service reported to Congress that it had found the highest radiation level in a television set to be 80,000 mr per hour, which is *1.6 million times* the acceptable safety level. The older a television set, the more radiation it is apt to give off. How safe is *your* television set?

Representative Paul Rogers (D-Fla.), coauthor of the Radiation Control Act, said at this time, "We brought him [Ott] to Washington for a briefing, but we didn't say anything for a while. We were afraid we would scare a lot of people. And when we checked the U.S. Surgeon General, he told us there was nothing to *worry* about."

Thank God for worriers. Dr. Ott is really worrying about us. As recently as October 1977, Dr. Ott told me that Representative Rogers has agreed to reopen the subject of television radiation for further investigation. I asked Dr. Ott what progress had been made since 1967. He told me that safety factors varied greatly with different sets, but that over the past four or five years each year there has been an increased number of sets recalled because of excess radiation.

One thing is sure. The more months a television tube is used, the more X-ray radiation is emitted. Another discomforting bit of news is that a color set has three "cathode guns," whereas black and white has but one. Net result? Viewers get *three times* as much radiation from color televsion as from black and white.

Dr. Ott's research has proved that radiation comes out of a television set in *all* directions. In one test case in Florida parents saw no change in their daughter's hyperkinetic behavior. The parents would not turn on the television until the little girl had gone to bed, but Dr. Ott found the problem. Her bed was in the next room, but her head was within a few feet of the set. Even though a wall was between her and the television set, she still got the effects. When the television set was moved, she improved.

In Ott's original television-exposed-rat experiments, sterility developed in rats *two rooms* away. These nonparticipating rats were in the primary "line of fire" from the television set. A safe distance from the set would be hard to determine.

Marie Franke, one of my laboratory technicians, told me an interesting story a few weeks ago. She and another technician were working with radioisotopes in a laboratory in Denver. They had worked with "wet isotopes" for years, and neither had ever had a positive reading on her radiation exposure badge. One month her friend's badge showed a dangerous level of exposure. The funny thing was, she was on vacation at the time. On the first day of vacation she dropped her brand new badge on the television set. During vacation she had watched television. On the last day of vacation she took the badge off the television set and turned it in for the next month's badge. The only place the badge could have gotten its exposure was the television set.

The way out? Yes, one way is to throw away the television. Might as well throw away the kids. Dr. Ott has designed a way out, but to my knowledge it is not available yet. He has designed the John Ott Box. This is a box that the television set slips into so that the set points straight up. Lead or other metal shielding protects the viewers from radiation, and they watch the image as reflected in a large mirror. He has a protective design for original sets, but of course the manufacturers would have to admit a problem existed if they adopted it. It probably wouldn't harm kids a whole lot to miss out on some of the 18,000 murders psychologists tell us they see before they begin school, and it might stir up a little creative imagination, but I foresee the John Ott Box as the only practical "way out."

Drugs. I would love to write a book and title it *Can't I Just Take a Pill?* (The answer is so obvious that the book probably wouldn't sell.) Don't we wish it were that kind of world. I am reminded of a patient who got really wide-eyed when I told him how high his cholesterol and triglycerides were. "Can't I do something about it—like smoke more?" Well, Howard, I wish it were true. I'd like to keep my weight under control by eating more, but . . . Can't I just take a pill? I think by now you may be getting the idea that we manufacture a lot of our own problems. If we really want to help our kids, it may require some lifestyle adjustments. But do it as a family improvement project, not as a jail sentence."

Just what do pills do for the hyperkinetic? I have heard caffeine recommended to calm the hyperkinetic kid. I have checked several drug reactions books and can't even find caffeine listed. That's strange because caffeine *is* a drug—an alkaloid—same family as codeine, morphine and nicotine. It *is* addicting (although socially acceptable) and *does* upset the body's chemistry. Some nutritionists say coffee is good food because it doesn't have any *calories*. No calories, but the havoc it can render! I have seen caffeine effects in literally thousands of people's chemistries. Giving you the results of my own observations and not so much textbook, these are the things I see:

There are six basic blood tests that respond when we consume caffeine. These are calcium, phosphorous, glucose, cholesterol, triglycerides, and uric acid. Let's look at them one at a time first, then in groups. These are the potential reactions in the blood:

Calcium is elevated. Result: Calcium can precipitate out of the blood and do damage where it deposits.

Phosphorous is lowered. Result: You are more susceptible to dental decay and other degenerative diseases.

Glucose is elevated. Result: This creates the potential for diabetes and heart disease, and is step one toward most degenerative diseases.

Cholesterol is elevated. Result: The low density lipoprotein portion of the cholesterol is elevated, which makes you a higher-risk candidate for heart attacks.

Triglycerides are elevated. Result:	This is seen as low-density lipoproteins and increases your risk of heart attack.
Uric Acid is elevated. Result:	Cause or effect? This condition is found in people with heart disease, arthritis, gum disease and other degenerative diseases.

Not *all* of these changes will be found in a single person at one time, but the *potential* for all of them is there when you take caffeine.

Now let's look at groups. Calcium and phosphorous combine together to form a compound which the body uses in building and maintaining strong bones and teeth. If the serum calcium goes up and the serum phosphorous goes down, there will be extra calcium, which will deposit somewhere. In dentistry it is seen as calcium deposits on the teeth, called calculus, or tartar. There is reason to believe the same imbalance can be the source of calcium that gets deposited in arthritic joints and in damaged vessels as arteriosclerosis. Wherever calcium deposits, it is not advantageous.

Elevated blood-sugar (glucose) levels are found in most of the degenerative diseases. Diabetes, of course, is the most notable, but even blood-sugar levels at the upper end of the "normal" range have been noted in gum diseases, dental decay and several medical diseases. As the glucose approaches an "ideal" point, most of these diseases show improvement. This does not imply that caffeine is the *sole* cause of these diseases, but it does mean that it works against the task of restoring a good chemical balance. If there are other things in the body—as from foods or drugs—that upset the same chemistry, then things begin to compound and disease can result.

Elevated cholesterol, triglycerides and uric acid in the blood have all been implicated in contributing to heart disease. Caffeine is a good elevator of all of these chemistries. Dietary fats don't compare to caffeine's ability to elevate the serum fats, cholesterol and triglycerides.

The uric acid level indicates the body's ability to metabolize proteins, and an elevation here is noted quickly by life insurance companies. The higher the uric acid, the higher the insurance premiums. What does all this lead up to? What should be a familiar concept by now. It creates the imbalance in the autonomic nervous system that we have been learning to balance throughout this book.

* * *

Addicting kids to caffeine while they are young does not appeal to me as a treatment for the hyperkinetic. What about Ritalin? For at least ten years Ritalin has been the treatment of choice for the hyperkinetic child. Who asks about its side-effects?—Daphne Roe, MD, a professor at Cornell University. In her *Drug-Induced Nutritional Deficiencies,* she tells about Ritalin. I don't recommend the book for the lay person because of its chemical complexity. It is very carefully written from the legal standpoint; the author uses chemical names for the drugs involved. Hence to find out what Ritalin does, first one must know that its chemical name is methylphenidate. It's pretty safe disguise, but I can see why she needed the protection. If the book were "translated into English," it could cause lots of problems with the drug industry.

In her section on Ritalin, Dr. Roe mentions that several researchers reported that "when hyperactive children are given stimulant drugs to control their behavior, initial weight loss occurs, this weight loss being usually only of transitory duration. That was in 1969. By 1972 more kids were receiving more Ritalin for longer periods and another study in 1972 showed that not only was there less weight, but less growth in height as well. If the drugged kids were taken off Ritalin during the summer they usually grew faster than average for the 3 months, then when school and drugs were resumed in the fall, growth was retarded again. For those kids who stayed on the drug during the summer there was little hope of catching up." Stunted growth—overgrowth—Stunted growth—what kind of development is this? Can't I just take a pill? Yes, if you are willing *to pay the price.*

The Reverend Chuck Aycock is one of those fellows who can turn a boy into a man in 10 days or your money back. I don't suppose he uses that slogan, but I feel that way about him. He is a bit more subtle in his approach. I saw him a few weeks back and told him of my excitement at nearing completion of *Why Raise Ugly Kids?* "Hold on a minute," he said with his eyes twinkling out from under his mountaineer hat. This trip he had about 70 kids from Michigan in tow. He was teaching them rock climbing and how to successfully battle the rapids in mountain streams. "Don't you finish that book until you have read Dr. Jim Dobson's book *Hide or Seek.*"

I've known Chuck long enough to know that he never wastes anyone's time. I bought the book. Yes, Chuck, I see why. Dr. Dobson has a perfect addition to *Why Raise Ugly Kids?* So far, we have talked about sleeping habits, foods, allergies, hyperkinetics, and a bunch of other things, but after all this is said and done, what *really* gets the kid launched into today's world? What's the spark that ignites the launch from childhood to adulthood? The feeling of *being* someone, the feeling of self-esteem. If you have all the health in the world going for you and you aren't someone of value to yourself, then life's a dud. Where does self-esteem come from? From parents, the same source that can also develop *lack* of self-esteem. Pretty important job, parenting.

Dr. Dobson points out that we live in a warped society. One that caters to the biggest, the strongest, the prettiest, to number one—especially in physical appearance. Somehow we get the idea that the only kids that count are those who can compose symphonies at age five, be the world's best quarterback, play chess blindfolded, but *never* come in second. Dr. Dobson says to this, "To the contrary, the vast majority of our children are not dazzlingly brilliant, extremely witty, highly coordinated, tremendously talented, or universally popular. They are just plain kids with oversized needs to be loved and accepted as they are. All kids may not be created equal, but they are all created worthy of the right to personal respect and dignity."

In his book, Dobson tells a story about a five-year-old girl. This story sums up our society's feelings toward physical appearance. By no outstanding achievement of her own she was born pretty, outstandingly so. He tells of how people who didn't know her would remark about what a cute child she was. That's not too hard to take, but then one day temporary tragedy struck. Dobson didn't describe it as tragedy, but then he isn't a dentist. A table and a front tooth met for an instant. Whomp! The little girl's tooth got displaced up into the bone and her lip swelled up in a peculiar fashion. The result didn't look like an accident—more like a birth defect. For the next few days she became transparent to passersby. People tried to pretend they didn't see the poor, deformed child. Her beauty was marred for a few days, but the reaction from an unknowing public was instantaneous and complete.

Dobson goes on to discuss the problems of placing too much emphasis on beauty, strength, winning first place only, etc., and points out the things that are of low priority on most kids' lists these days. These included honesty, integrity, courage, craftsmanship, humor, motherhood, loyalty, patience and diligence. Where do kids develop value systems for things like these? Military academies? Try home. Dr. Dobson gives ideas of how to incorporate these things into the minds of our growing kids. What could be of more value? How do you speak about your child to other adults in the kid's presence? "Oh, he's just like his father—never finishes anything he starts." How will he grow up? Does he really have a choice? Will he "never finish anything" or will he pick that up as a *challenge* and "show the world?" His self-esteem is what makes the difference.

A few days after finishing the first chapter of Dobson's *Hide or Seek,* I raced for a plane whose schedule had been moved forward five minutes. I clambered aboard the plane as the first engine was screaming its disappointment at being awakened and clumsily made my way to my seat. I was carrying a portable public address system in one hand, my briefcase in the other, and a two-wheeled trolly under my arm. I *would* get the middle seat. That meant that the fellow on the aisle had to get up while I put my six-foot frame into a five-foot space and juggled my carry-on items while removing my coat. What does one do when he is performing ungracefully in front of 50 passengers who have nothing better to do than stare blankly at his struggles? To maintain sanity he smiles and says a few funny words to the nearby viewers. I smiled at the 19-year-old girl in the window seat and said, "It would sure be easier if I had one less leg." She smiled an understanding smile and helped me slip the P.A. system under her seat space. "I really appreciate that," I said. It was sure going to be crowded with all my stuff. Now she had a frown on her face as if she didn't comprehend my babbling. Then I noticed that she was pointing to both of her ears and shaking her head. She couldn't hear. She was deaf. I nodded, smiled, looked straight ahead and prepared to get interested in the flight magazine. Then it hit me. There was the little girl Jim Dobson was telling about. Not really, but look at the situation. She's "different." How easy it would be to ignore her. And without hurting her feelings, for by age 19 I am sure many people had chosen silence as a copout.

I turned to her and asked with careful enunciation, "Can you read lips?"

"A little bit," she mouthed back.

I reached into my briefcase, pulled out a large writing pad that always accompanies me on long trips. "Where are you going?" I wrote.

"To Michigan to school. I'm going to learn to be a medical technologist."

"I saw something on television a few days ago about a special school for deaf people. Is this where you are going?"

"No—a regular school."

"Your folks live in Colorado Springs?"

Within a few minutes this little gal was writing as fast as anyone I have ever seen. She told me all kinds of things about her parents' background, her aspirations in college, her plans afterwards—and all of a sudden we were in Chicago. Somehow I felt protective and responsible for her.

"What airline from here?" I wrote.

"American."

"Me too. Let's walk over together."

She grinned acceptance.

Once we got to American's concourse I panicked. There was no gate listing for her flight and mine was near departure. Surely she could take care of herself—but in that world of silence? I asked an American employee when the gate announcement would be up. "Oh, I'm a stewardess on that flight." I explained my concern that my deaf friend might miss her flight, and the stewardess very politely said, "Don't worry, I'll take her there myself. It's just down the concourse and the announcement will be up on the screen shortly." As the two women walked away I felt a wave of emotion. I could so easily have ignored her, but by recognizing her as an individual I found what a world of silence *I* lived in. It was as if I had just had a deep personal experience with God. I had stepped over a social threshold and found a new world—one so many people are self-excluded from. All this pent up inside me in a brief moment as I hesitated before entering my plane. Two warm tears raced down my left cheek and my eyes grew blurry for an instant. The man next to me was watching. "Your daughter?" he asked.

"No," I answered, "I don't even know her name."

Chapter Twelve

How to Tell Your Children About Good Nutrition

How do you get the family to work with you? There are ways, and it is easier on everyone when you know them. Joannie Huggins shares some techniques of harmony and hunger in the home.

Most books written by married men are dedicated to their wives. This is probably an act of appeasement because it "takes time away from the family" to write books. My book is dedicated to the memory of Harvey Stallard because it is the fruit of a seed he planted. Besides, this book didn't take me away from my family. It brought me to them—well, her.

Now that the kids are gone, the major disturbance in our once noisy house is the cat yawning. When I am at home there are many disturbances in the form of telephone calls to be returned, letters to be answered, patients to be seen and visitors to be entertained. When I write, my wife Joanie and I go off to some secluded oceanside cabin. By choice we seldom eat out. My lecture schedule provides plenty of restaurants. We do something we never do at home. We go to bed when we are tired, and get up when we are rested. We jog along the ocean for however long we want, eat when hungry, and write until the words stop. We then seek nonwriting-oriented adventures. Because home is in the mountains, the slightest form of sea life becomes an adventure. Tides are meaningful. I try to conceive of the volume of water that moves when the tide comes out. How big a vat would it fill if suspended in the sky? I've only seen one living blue crab—right in the middle of chapter six.

We write and play. It's the most fun we have all year—and probably the most productive.

Last year when I asked Joanie to write up some really good-tasting recipes for a cookbook for my patients, she undertook the task of writing down a few dozen. By the end of the year she had a cookbook nearly 500 pages long. Was she put upon? She doesn't think so. It went into its third printing within six months and is distributed by all kinds of people. A furniture store in Virginia buys 20 copies every six weeks; a high school home economics class in Colorado is using her book as a guide for cooking classes. She's part of the team. She has now sold nearly 50,000 copies.

She's also good at giving mothers suggestions on how to incorporate good nutrition ideas into daily living. I've asked her to tell you about two of her favorite subjects: how to involve the kids in good nutrition habits and what to do with the picky eater.

This is Joanie's chapter.

While lecturing with my husband across the country, I often hear the same question from mothers: "How do I tell my children about nutrition and body chemistry so they're with me and not fighting me?" Here are some suggestions for parents on how to present the concept of healthful living to the whole family. It is important to have the family unit interested and supportive of the parents' efforts to bring the best possible foods into the home.

What we are really talking about is an economic issue—how to squeeze the most value from our food budget. Some gals are super smart—they spend money on good nutrition instead of spending the family's money on junk food their children want. There is just so much money allocated to spend on food; now let's take a look at how smart, nutrition-conscious, dollar-wise parents spend their food dollars.

We are all on a food budget of some kind, and it is each family's responsibility to get the best possible nutrients for each food dollar spent. Whenever I go to the supermarket I am saddened by the wasted food dollars I see mothers spending. Take potatoes, for instance. They are about 10 cents a pound raw. Made into potato chips they are $1.25 a pound. These potato chips are empty calories, very few nutrients and mostly calories. Soda pop costs about $5.98 a case, and often I see three cases of pop in a shopping cart for a family for a week.

This is what I'm talking about when I say "empty calories," because these families are spending a large percentage of their weekly food budgets on calories with no nutrients. Fifteen ounces of cream-filled snacks sell for $1.43. That's $1.53 per pound of sugar-filled, additive-laden, teeth-rotting calories—with very little nutrient. Read the label the next time you buy one of these snack packets and see what you are giving your children. You could buy a lot of fresh fruit and vegetables on what you are spending for this junk food. You could also buy a lot of 100 percent whole-grain bread and peanut butter with this "wasted" money. Nutrients are what the body uses to rebuild tissues. This rebuilding is done on a daily basis. Many mothers tell me that it actually costs less when they buy good food—fresh vegetables, fruits, nuts and meat—because the "empty-calorie" foods are by far the most expensive. In the long run, they are doubly expensive because of the high volume of sugar in most of them—meaning more dental bills because sugar rots teeth.

The families that have had the most success with presenting a good dietary plan to their children have been very honest with the children regarding the food budget. Children are quick to pick up on budgets and what it takes to make them work: careful planning. These families have involved their children of *all* ages in food buying and preparation.

Toddlers can help stir the oatmeal, cornmeal mush, scrambled eggs, cookie and cake batter, and watch the egg timers. They can draw and color place mats for the family, make posters of good foods to eat, make centerpieces for the table and fold the napkins. They can also make special table decorations for birthdays and holidays. Little ones get a sense of great personal value when they are contributing to the family meals. Take a picture of your toddler stirring oatmeal and display it in a prominent place. Stick it on the refrigerator. We are really talking about the child's self-esteem, so fragile at times and in need of recognition. When you involve the entire family in this business of food buying and preparation you are giving each member a sense of self-worth and recognition. Try it. It works!

When you are talking to the family about changing eating habits—getting sugar, white flour, additives and preservatives out of the diet—

keep the discussion upbeat, never hangdog. For instance, don't say "We are giving up white bread." Instead say "We are changing to foods that give us the most nutrients and food value for our money." When you do decide to change your eating and buying habits, try not to "preach" about it to everyone. You most likely will find yourself an "outsider," maybe left out of parties and activities because you are so "preachy" and hung up on what you're doing. You *are* on the right track (you *know* you are), but no one is really interested. So do it quietly and maybe a little deviously!

Let the preschoolers set the table and clean up after meals to teach them responsibility. Should parents be servants? Children can and should be taught to clean up their kitchen messes. Let them make granola and wheat sticks, stuff the celery, cut the cheese, tear the salad greens and pour the salad dressing. Preschoolers can make their own recipe book by cutting out pictures of foods they help prepare. They take such pride in this! This is really behavior modification by giving recognition and approval for tasks well performed. This way you also are making food buying and preparation of more value to your family by giving it more importance.

Let preschoolers pick out the serving dishes to use. Pretty and unusual dishes can be bought for next to nothing at garage sales and flea markets, and children love to choose which one to use at each meal. Who says everything has to match? I have bought some really pretty and unusual baskets for 25 cents at flea markets. Some I spray-painted and used for nuts, salads and whole-grain crackers or cookies. Sometimes I line them with foil and bright napkins and serve all the makings for building hamburgers—pickles, olives, tomatoes, lettuce, sprouts, cucumbers, onions and whole-wheat hamburger buns. What a festive table it is when you use baskets, and so inexpensive when you buy them at flea markets!

Another fun thing to do is to encourage school-age children to look in the town library for books on colonial American eating habits. They can also discuss recipes the pioneers made and try them in your home for a special dinner, with everyone participating in the food preparation.

This opens up the opportunity to discuss the subject of good manners. Let the preschoolers draw and color pictures of children using both good and bad table manners. Have a lively discussion with the whole family about the duties of host and hostess (invitations, food preparation and serving, cleaning house, dressing up, greeting guests and seeing that they are comfortable). You should also discuss the duties of a guest (arrive on time, never bring personal problems to the party, dress up, offer to help, offer some interesting conversation, leave at an appropriate hour, send a thank-you note or phone a message of thanks). Plan a small dinner party with friends and have each family member perform his assigned task. This way children get the idea that parties are a family affair; you will help with their parties, and they will help with yours. One of the best summer parties we've gone to was one where the children were cooking the chicken on the grill and making homemade ice cream.

One evening my husband and I were invited out to some friends' home for dinner. Their ten-year-old son, George, loved to help with meal service. When the wine was served, guess who came to the table with a clean white towel over his arm and a chilled wine bottle in his hand? George, of course! He showed my husband the label, uncorked the bottle, set the cork down for my husband to examine, then poured a small amount in his glass and stepped back. He was as professional as the finest wine steward in the country. He did a fine job and was silently proud of his accomplishment, as he should have been.

Buy inexpensive and different egg cups at the dime store and let the kids pick out the cups they want to use this day (for soft-boiled eggs). Soft-boiled eggs for breakfast served in each family member's own egg cup probably take the least amount of time for a busy mother and have the most nutrients. Let each family member "do" his own egg. Slice off the very top of the soft-boiled egg (sitting in its egg cup) with a knife and eat the contents with a spoon. Easy for mom and super nutritious for the family.

Make a list of interesting foods to talk about at dinner and have a food-of-the-week discussion one night each week at the dinner table. Talk about the different ways to cook the food (bake, steam, broil, microwave), how best to store it (can it, freeze it, dry it), how it is grown and where.

One of the best ways to give value and status to food buying and preparation is to let the children do it. I have seen children as young as eight years doing the weekly shopping at the supermarket by themselves. One woman in our seminar in California said she started her little girl at age six with four items to pick up and pay for while the mother waited outside in the car. The mother had cut out pictures of the things she wanted her daughter to buy, and the daughter knew the brands her mother wanted and where they were located in the supermarket. The mother told me she gave her daughter enough money to cover the cost of these foods. A few months later the daughter was able to buy more items, and by age eight she was doing all the grocery shopping by herself. Children love to be given this responsibility. Children make good comparison shoppers, so give them the opportunity. This takes careful planning at first. For instance, if whole chicken is on special and no one in your family likes dark meat, then it's not a special for your family. Children usually make better comparison shoppers than parents because they have more time, they are proud of their shopping talents, and they don't want the privilege taken away. Of course, a few mistakes will be made, but haven't we all made some lulus? Be careful not to scold—especially in the beginning—next week will be better. Have the whole family become label readers, and if an item has sugar (dextrose, maltose, cane sugar, corn sugar) or additives or preservatives in it, leave it on the shelf.

The parents I know who are letting the children take over the weekly grocery shopping leave the kids alone at the supermarket and go off on other errands. Some parents give the kids enough cash to cover the weekly bill, others give a signed check made out to the supermarket. I would recommend talking with the manager and telling him what you are doing so there will be no surprises for the children who have a check. We are talking about the greatest gift you can give your child—building his self-esteem.

A very big bonus happens when the kids come home with the groceries. They get to put them away. What a bear carrying in the groceries and putting them away has always been for mothers. What a blessing it is when all the children know where everything goes in the kitchen and what a help this is to a busy mother!

Why not have a team of two family members take turns cooking Sunday dinner? Vary the combination so it won't be the same two working together all the time.

The families I know where the children have been doing the grocery shopping and helping with the food preparation settle into routines as far as talents go. Each family member knows how to do all things—make soups and stew, grill, make salads, bake—but each kid tends to have his own area of expertise. One of the kids likes to bake best, another likes to make soups, another likes to grill, and each becomes expert in the area of his greatest interest.

One of the most appreciated gifts you can give your child is the ability to handle himself as an adult by age 18—in other words, *adult at 18.* By participating in food buying and preparation from early childhood, your child becomes well equipped to take care of his own needs and be a terrific parent himself when he marries and has his own children.

* * *

"What do you do when your kids won't eat?" This must be a common problem, judging from the number of times I am asked this question when my husband and I are giving a seminar. Here are some tips on how other mothers have handled this problem successfully.

The hardest thing for young mothers to accept is the fact that mother is usually the one responsible for a child's eating habits. I know that's difficult to take. But the feedback I received from parents who have tried the following suggestions leads me to believe the situation is not insurmountable.

The number one problem seems to be with vegetables. I can't really blame the kids for not liking them the way they are usually prepared—boiled to death, mushy and practically tasteless. This is *not* the way vegetables were intended to be served. They should be eaten raw or steamed for a few minutes so they are still crisp.

The toddler in the highchair can be served his vegetables first, when he's hungriest. You can cut up *raw* broccoli, cauliflower, string beans, lettuce and zucchini and let him eat these crunchy morsels first. Then comes the meat and then, *only* if everything is finished, some fresh fruit or wholesome whole-grain and sugar-free dessert. Children learn early how to beg, and parents all too often give in to them just to avoid a fuss. This puts the children in charge of the situation, and that is not good. Show them early with much love and firmness that *you* are in control and *you* will not accept whining and fussing as general behavior.

Another way successful mothers have to get their picky eaters to eat is to *never* give them between-meal snacks. Their little stomachs get full very quickly, and they simply cannot handle snacks and regular meals too. Some mothers protest that a child is hungry and can't wait for the next meal. Poor little creature, he will certainly starve to death. You see, the child has been carefully taught that he doesn't have to eat this meal. He'll keep getting snacks because mother feels sorry for him. Believe me, your child will eat his meals if he gets hungry enough. There are very few cases of voluntary starvation recorded. I never allowed any snacks, and I never had any picky eaters either. By snacks, I mean food of any kind, and milk. Soon after milk hits the stomach it becomes solid, and then picky eaters aren't hungry. Don't give any juice one hour before a meal. Limit all liquids at mealtime also, so the kids won't fill up on milk and juices. If they are thirsty, give them water. You might be amazed at how much of the food budget is spent on juices, drinks and pop. We are the only society that drinks so much juice and pop. We push juice on our kids practically from their first month of life. Juice is expensive. Almost all juices have either sugar or chemicals added to them, and they are an expensive habit to push on our kids. If someone is thirsty, give him water. It's still the best thirst quencher.

It is best to avoid a confrontation over eating habits. Simply, lovingly and firmly refuse to accept fussing and begging from the children. Ignore it. They soon learn you aren't listening! If I were given the task of retraining a picky eater—a child who had learned early that fussing and begging would get him anything he wanted, a child who knew he didn't have to eat at mealtime because he could wheedle all the snacks he wanted out of mother—if I were given this task today, this is what I'd do:

I would set a pretty place for him for breakfast, as usual. After about 20 minutes, if he were just playing around with his food, I would clear the table off without any comment. I would not scold (I know this part is hard, but it's an investment). After about an hour I know he's going to come asking for a snack. When he does, I would gently and firmly tell him that lunch will be served at noon, and if he is still hungry, he can eat then. I would not give him *any* snacks or juice, just water. At lunch I would again set a pretty place and give him about 20 minutes to eat it. Then, again with no hassle, clear the table. Again, *no* snacks at all until dinner. It usually takes one or two days for kids to find out you mean business about their snacking. When they eat their meals properly, I might start giving them *very small* snacks of dried fruit and nuts when they are hungry, but *only* if they continue to eat well at mealtime.

I would also serve meals in different areas. They don't always have to be eaten at the table. Have a picnic outside, or if it rains, on a plastic tablecloth on the living room floor. How about in front of a roaring fire in the fireplace? I do not recommend a picky eater eating in front of the television. It's too distracting. If you have been using television as a babysitter during meals, maybe that's the problem. Television offers too many distractions for little minds that are supposed to be thinking about eating.

I would give the little picky eater a reward every time he cleaned his plate—a piece of fruit or a whole-grain cookie, never anything that contains processed sugar.

If all these suggestions are followed, your picky-eater problem may be solved within a week. That's a small investment for years of returns.

Chapter Thirteen

How to Raise Beautiful Brats

Putting it all together

Stallard's original challenge to me was to find a way to "package" babies. Well, after all this preliminary study I figured I was as ready as I would ever be, so I attacked the problem with some paper, a pencil, and a pair of scissors. With the aid of scotch tape I came up with a paper design of a modern cradleboard. If it's modern it should have a modern name, one that describes what it does. It helps develop proper faces and helps develop proper bodies skeletally. Orthodontics and orthopedics. It also sleeps kids. Therefore "Orthocrib" was born. After much fuss and trial in the design phase, I decided I was ready to make one. Molds were pretty expensive but could be made out of hydrocal. Hydrocal is a plaster that I work with daily. I figured the mold would weigh about 100 pounds, but what can you mix 100 pounds of plaster in—especially when you consider the more volume you have the faster it sets? A four-ounce mix will set in less than five minutes. At that rate, 100 pounds would probably set in seconds.

Somehow I conned my assistant, technician and receptionist into mixing plaster and washing bowls. I built the mold for the Orthocrib, then we started mixing plaster. Well, that 100 pounds gets pretty warm when you are adding four ounces at a time, and the setting time goes faster. By the time we were halfway through, the plaster was setting within 15 seconds of the time it hit the form. Faster! We had to mix, spread and wash faster. Ten seconds, then eight seconds. We all began to sweat. By the time I topped off the form, the plaster was setting when it touched the mass of steamy imitation rock. It had taken 32 fast-moving minutes, but we made it.

Little did I realize that was the easy part. I soon found out why molds cost so much. That weekend I started chiseling with hammers and tools. By Saturday afternoon I could see that weekend project would extend into months. Hydrocal is hard. Steeped in training of the modern world, I drove to town and rented a power sander. That was the answer—to black lung disease. I'll never get it. Mine are too full of white plaster to let anything else get in. You can't imagine the mess. It was like a heavy, warm snowfall. When the light grew faint I knew I had better quit. Have you ever seen an all-white dental laboratory? I had one. It took three days of scrubbing to get to the point of repainting the room, but I had an Orthocrib mold.

How close did it approximate a baby's backside? I didn't know. I have a patient named Connie. The last time I had seen her she was—to put it her way—"with child." I called her to check her with-without-child status and found that she now had a two-month-old son.

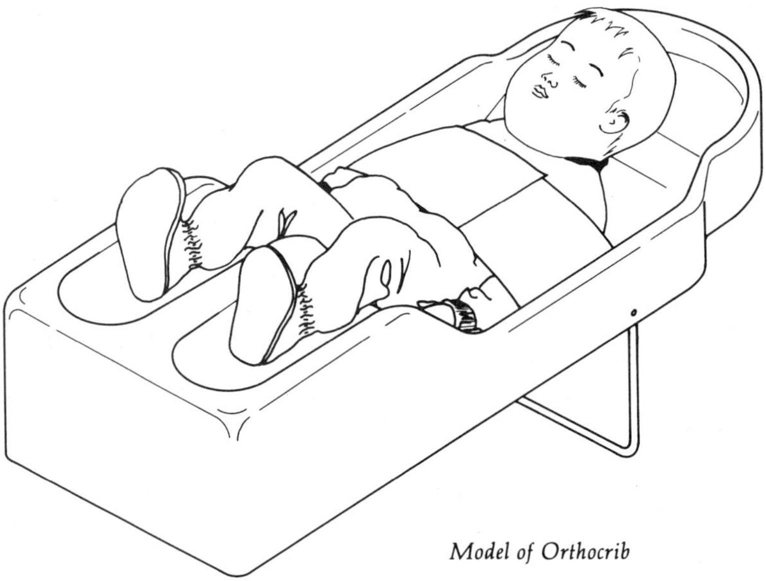

Model of Orthocrib

"Can I borrow his butt?" I asked.

"For posterity or posteriority?" she quipped.

Walt was not really interested in science, especially when it included lying on cold plaster. After a little chiseling and lots of baby talk the mold fit much better.

Plastic selection, hinges for the back, swaddling bands—all these things finally came together and I had a package to show Harvey. I had a package that protected the head from side bumps, held the back straight, held the shoulder blades flat, swaddled the arms, but left the legs free. Velcro allowed for individual fitting of the swaddling band. The bottom half of the Orthocrib was elevated so that the legs rested at about a 35-degree angle to the body, giving the hips the best opportunity for proper development. Legs separated, knees elevated, back straight, no hands, arms, thumbs or pillows around the face—what more could Harvey ask?

Harvey had not heard about my studies for over six months, but as program chairman of the International Academy of Gnathology, he had asked me to give a 30-minute presentation on my findings. I found out later that he thought I had spent maybe a week on the subject. Was he surprised! Now it was his turn to cry. He had no idea that I had amassed so much information substantiating what he had been suggesting for 45 years. I've known Harvey to be speechless once. This was the time. I was virtually unknown to the gathered 500 men that Friday morning. I was to be "on" at 11:30. The man sitting next to me had attended a course I was attending the year before, but he couldn't remember my name. At 11:20 he picked up the program schedule, wrinkled his nose, muttered "sleeping habits," and turned to me.

"Know this guy?"

"Yes."

"Any good?"

"Quite good."

"Think I'll cut out and play tennis. Rather do that than eat lunch anyway."

"Oh, I think you should stay. Bet you'll like it. You'll probably hear things you've never heard at a dental meeting before."

"Well, if you think it's *that* good, I'll stay."

At that moment the introduction was over, and I rose, shook hands with my red-faced friend, and walked to the speakers' platform. He knows my name now.

Thirty minutes later Harvey was on cloud nine. His 45-year-old baby had come to life. He couldn't believe it. That evening at the banquet Harvey came over to me at salad time and said he wanted to introduce me to some people. An hour and fifteen minutes later he deposited me in front of my drooping ice cream dessert. Something was missing in between, but Harvey had just introduced me to over 100 people who would later become close friends and add immensely to my knowledge of the treatment of oral diseases. I had done what Harvey asked. I thought I was finished. How could I be so wrong? I was only beginning.

* * *

What if you're bigger than a baby? How do you change the sleeping habits of someone over a year old? Actually, it's easy—up to age 21, then it's *really* tough. First, of course, you must have interest. We do this through education. We tell our patients about beautiful faces and bodies if they are girls, and if they are boys we talk about sports advantages if both halves of the body develop equally. To both we mention speed of orthodontic treatment and the possibilities of relapse. If old habits are not corrected, you can wear a retainer for 10 years and still have a relapse when it is removed if "outside" pressure is still there.

The technique part is simple, easy, fast and highly successful. What more could you ask? We tell the kids: "When you go to bed, lie on your back for 10 minutes. [Usually, the kid is asleep in 10 minutes, but putting it this way doesn't sound restricting.] If you haven't fallen asleep, then stand on your ear or anything that feels comfortable. When Mom and Dad go to bed, they are going to come in and flip you over on your back. This kinda wakes you up a bit, but you'll know what they are doing and go back to sleep. The folks will get up before you do in the morning and flip you over again. Usually, after a week of doing this you will be a back sleeper."

It seldom takes more than this to develop the habit, and rarely will someone revert to old habits after the new one is established. If additional "therapy" is required, a sleeping bag can be used. Put the sleeping bag on the bed and let the child sleep in it. The "mummy-case" type is best, for it is really hard to sleep in any position *but* on your back in one of these.

What about pillows? Harvey has a bunch of pictures of pillows of the world. They are many and varied, but most of them are designed for back sleeping. One of the best I have seen is made from two washcloths sewn together. A one-inch slot is left in one end, then foam (polyurethane is good) can be stuffed in the hole. After it's full, sew it up. Doubled over, this makes an excellent pillow for keeping the back (spine) straight and supporting the head.

* * *

Well, what have we got? A new child culture. One devoted to the development of "beautiful brats." Harvey's original ideas set me to investigating and evaluating many child cultures. What I have compiled pulls the best of those worlds together in support of his original concepts.

It all starts with the twinkle in Daddy's eye—maybe even before. It is as true today as in centuries gone by that it takes healthy parents to give birth to healthy kids. Three, six, nine months prior to conception—does it really matter? The important thing to remember is to be healthy all the time during your potential childbearing years. Good health is still your best investment. You don't have to reserve it just for the kid's sake—enjoy it yourself.

So while you're young and growing strong and taking hold the reins,
Take care to watch of what you eat, what runs within your veins . . .

If you know several months in advance of a pregnancy, then by all means, stick to the suggestions of adequate carbohydrates, fat and protein, with special emphasis on vitamins and minerals. If a little bit's good, then a lot is worse than nothing. Don't overdo.

Do watch out for drugs. Just because it's not a prescription item doesn't mean it's safe for your child. Now and then we all get headaches. Okay, so take aspirin, but not for a month. Can't sleep? Reread the section on honey. Sleeping pills—even the mild ones—are not going to help produce better kids. Your body can tolerate two or three of most anything, but may not tolerate the self-medication, taken daily for weeks on end. If you are really hooked on some mild nonprescription or prescription medication, express your concern to your obstetrician and let him help you.

Caffeine is now hitting the newspapers as a no-no for pregnancy. You know about sugar and other endocrine disturbers so take heed, or

. . . should we fail to do our part, the upkeep and the rent,
The landlord has his time of grace, then out of shape gets bent.

By following these suggestions, I wish for you that you may: give your kids the maximum greatness bound up in *your* heredity; learn to package them and sleep them in such a manner to give them bilaterally balanced bodies; feed them right; avoid things that create the hyperkinetic kid; and build them boundless self-esteem so they will

Learn what to do to pull you through, and when to ply the skids,
Cause no one wants the lousy task of raising Ugly Kids.

Bibliography

Aikawa, Jerry K., MD. *The Relationship of Magnesium to Disease in Domestic Animals and In Humans.* Springfield, Illinois: Charles C. Thomas, 1971.

Boaz, Franz. *Cradles of the Kwakiutl Indians.* American Museum of Natural History, Memoir, 8:458460.

Bureau of American Ethnology. "Artificial Head Deformation." *A-M Handbook of American Indians,* Bulletin 30, part I.

———. *Handbook of American Indians.* Taylor Museum, 1912.

Cheraskin, Emanuel. "Effect of Carbohydrate Supplements Upon the Height of the T-wave in Lead I" *Angiology,* April 1968.

———. "Total Health, A Correlative Study in Stomatology and Electrocardiology. "*Annals of Dentistry,* Spring 1979.

Cheraskin, Emanuel et al. *Diet and Disease.* Emmaus, Pennsylvania: Rodale Books, 1968.

———. *Diet and the Periodontal Patient.* Springfield, Illinois: Charles C. Thomas, 1970.

Delacato, Carl H. *The Diagnosis and Treatment of Speech and Reading Problems.* Springfield, Ill.: Charles C. Thomas, 1963.

———. *A New Start for the Child with Reading Problems.* New York: McKay, 1970.

———. *The Ultimate Stranger: The Autistic Child.* Garden City, N.Y.: Doubleday, 1974.

Dennis, Wayne. "Cradles and Cradling Practices of the Pueblo Indians." *American Anthropologist,* 42: 107–15, 1940.

Dobson, James. *Hide or Seek.* Old Tappan, New Jersey: Revell Publishing Company.

Doman, Glenn J. *How to Teach Your Baby to Read: The Gentle Revolution.* New York: Random House, 1964.

———. *Teach Your Baby Math.* New York: Simon and Schuster, 1979.

———. *What to Do About Your Brain Injured Child.* Garden City, N.Y.: Doubleday, 1974.

Fluhrer, A. Vernon. "Some Original Investigations into Pressure Habits as Etiological Factors in Dentofacial Abnormalities." *American Journal of Orthodontics,* 36: 37–57, 1950.

Greenacre, Phyllis. "Infant Reactions to Restraint; Problems in the Fate of Infantile Agression." *American Journal of Orthospsychiatry,* 14: 204–18, April, 1944.

Huggins, Hal A. "Two Faces of Cholesterol." *Chicago Dental Society Review.* 68:22–29, January 1975.

Huggins, Joanie. *Out of the Sugar Rut.* Colorado Springs, Colorado: HAH Publications, 1978.

Jacobson, Alexander. "Thumbsucking; a Psychological and Dental Understanding of the Problem." *International Journal of Orthodontics,* December 1962.

Jarvis, D.C., MD. *Arthritis and Folk Medicine.* Greenwich, Conn.: Fawcett, 1960.

Kalokerinos, Archie. *Every Second Child.* Nashville, Tenn.: Thomas Nelson, 1974.

Keith, Sir Arthur. *Menders of the Maimed.* London: Oxford University Press, 1919.

Kinderlehrer, Jane. *Cooking With Love and Wheat Germ.* Emmaus, Pennsylvania: Rodale Press, 1977.

Klein, Ernest T. "Pressure Habits, Etiological Factors in Malocclusion." *American Journal of Orthodontics,* 38: 8: 569–87, August 1952.

Mason, Otis T. "Cradles of American Aborigines." *U.S. National Museum Report,* pp. 161–212, 1887.

Oster, K. "Plasmologen Diseases—A New Concept of Etiology of Atherosclerosis." *American Journal of Clinical Research* 2: 30–35, 1971.

Ott, John N. *Health and Light.* Old Greenwich, Conn.: Devin-Adair, 1973.

Page, Melvin. *Degeneration-Regeneration.* Biochemical Research Foundation, 1949.

Pokrovsky, Egor A. *Physical Training of Children of Various Peoples in Primary Russia.* Society of Friends of Natural Science, vol. 45, 1866.

———. *Transactions of the Society of Friends of Natural Science and Anthropology,* vol. 14.

Price, Weston A. *Nutrition and Physical Degeneration.* La Mesa, California: Price-Pottenger Foundation, 1945.

Roe, Daphne A., MD. *Drug-Induced Nutritional Deficiencies.* AVI Publishing, 1976.

Ross, T. J., Stephen V. Sharnick, K. Oster. "Liposomes as a Proposed Vehicle for the Absorption of Bovine Xanthine Oxidase." *Proceedings of the Society for Experimental Biology in Medicine,* 163: 141–45, January 1980.

Schroeder, Henry A., MD. *The Trace Elements and Man.* Old Greenwich, Conn.: Devin-Adair, 1973.

Stallard, Harvey. "A Consideration of Extraoral Pressures in the Etiology of Malocclusions." *International Journal of Orthodontia, Oral Surgery and Radiography,* vol. XVI, no. 5, May 1930.

———. "The General Prevalence of Gross Symptoms of Malocclusion. *Dental Cosmos,* vol. 24:29–37, January 1932.

———. "The General Relation of Pillowing to Malocclusion." *Dental Cosmos,* March 1925.

Steinman, Ralph R., John Leonora, Department of Physiology and Biophysics, School of Medicine, and Department of Oral Medicine, Loma Linda University. *Evidence Suggesting the Existence of a Hypothalamic-Parotid Gland Endocrine Axis,* 83:807–15, October 1968.

Veras, Raymundo, David Melton, Glenn J. Doman. *Children of Dreams, Children of Hope.* Chicago: Regnery, 1975.

Verrett, Jacqueline. *Eating May be Hazardous to Your Health.* New York: Doubleday, 1975.

Vogel, Richard, DMD, et al. *"The Effect of Folic Acid on Ginggival Health."* *Journal of Periodontology,* 47:667, November 1976.

Watson, E. H., MD, and G. H. Lowrey, MD. *Growth and Development of Children.* Chicago: Year Book Publishers, 1954.

Whitman, Clifford L. "Habits Can Mean Trouble." *Washington State Dental Journal,* January 1952.

Index